REVIEW OF
PATHOLOGY

REVIEW OF
PATHOLOGY

SECOND EDITION

Ivan Damjanov, M.D., Ph.D.

Professor of Pathology
Department of Pathology
The University of Kansas School of Medicine
Kansas City, Kansas

Emanuel Rubin, M.D.

Gonzalo E. Aponte Professor and Chairman
Department of Pathology, Anatomy and Cell Biology
Jefferson Medical College
Thomas Jefferson University
Philadelphia, Pennsylvania

LIPPINCOTT WILLIAMS & WILKINS
A **Wolters Kluwer** Company
Philadelphia • Baltimore • New York • London
Buenos Aires • Hong Kong • Sydney • Tokyo

Editor: Paul J. Kelly
Managing Editor: Crystal Taylor
Marketing Manager: Christine Kushner
Project Editor: Jennifer D. Weir

351 West Camden Street
Baltimore, Maryland 21201-2436 USA

227 East Washington Square
Philadelphia, PA 19106

Printed in the United States of America

First Edition, 1994

Library of Congress Cataloging-in-Publication Data

Damjanov, Ivan.
   Review of pathology / Ivan Damjanov, Emanuel Rubin.—2nd ed.
     p.   cm.
   ISBN 0-397-58408-3 (paper)
   1. Pathology Examinations, questions, etc.   I. Rubin, Emanuel,
  1928–   . II. Title.
   [DNLM: 1. Pathology Examination Questions.   QZ 18.2 D161r 2000]
   RB31.D35   2000
   610.07′076—dc21
   DNLM/DCL   99-33310
   for Library of Congress   CIP

To purchase additional copies of this book, call our customer service department at **(800) 638-3030** or fax orders to **(301) 824-7390**. For other book services, including chapter reprints and large quantity sales, ask for the Special Sales department.

For all other calls originating outside of the United States, please call **(301) 714-2324**.

Visit Lippincott Williams & Wilkins on the Internet: **http://www.lww.com**. Lippincott Williams & Wilkins customer service representatives are available from 8:30 am to 6:00 pm, EST, Monday through Friday, for telephone access.

99 00 01 02 03
1 2 3 4 5 6 7 8 9 10

Preface

This review is designed to focus your attention on the most important facts and ideas that comprise the study of pathology and to assist you in relating these facts to an understanding of human disease. It includes chapters on both general and systemic pathology. The questions are presented in the formats used in standardized examinations. The answer sections will (1) show you the concepts that are illustrated by the questions, (2) point out the reasoning behind both the correct and the incorrect choices, and (3) explain the incorrect associations that may lead you to the wrong answer because of faulty logic or a lack of knowledge or the correct answer for the wrong reason.

The previous edition of our review was well received by students, and we are pleased that so many of them have given us feedback and suggestions on how to improve it. We have now done the following:

- *Shortened the book to make it more manageable.* To this end we have eliminated most of the questions considered by the former users to be "too detailed," "too esoteric," or "nonessential."
- *Made the questions more clinically relevant.* We have rewritten most of the questions from the previous edition and added some 400 new questions based on clinical vignettes. To answer these questions one needs a solid knowledge of pathology in a clinical context since the National Board of Medical Examiners (NBME) emphasizes the clinical relevance of pathology. In fact, approximately 70% of all pathology questions on the USMLE I are related to clinical findings or pathophysiology. Our new questions should provide students with a good preparation for the Boards.
- *Used only the question formats sanctioned by the NBME.* All the questions are now either in the *multiple-choice* format or in the form of *extended matching questions* (one correct out of 20 possibilities). Note that extended matching questions are a new format used by the NBME, and our book will provide students with an opportunity to practice appropriately. Furthermore, as you will realize yourself, *extended matching questions* are an excellent way of reviewing large amounts of material in a short period of time. We anticipate that these questions will be most popular before your final examinations and the USMLE I.

Toward the end of the book you will find a *comprehensive examination* designed to test your overall understanding of pathology. You should consider a score of 70% to be passing, and scores over 85% are outstanding. If you do not achieve a passing score on our final examination, you may not be well prepared for your own final or the USMLE-1. You should then review the subjects with which you had difficulty and test yourself again.

The last section of the book is a practical examination based on color photographs. Because color photographs figure prominently in standardized national examinations, the 24 pictorial questions provide you with an opportunity to test your interpretive skills. There is abundant information in the illustrations, and we encourage you to seek out their accompanying text discussions as part of your review.

Each of the more than 1000 questions in this book tests not only the fact that corresponds to the correct answer, but also two to four closely related concepts. Thus, this book covers about 3000 of the most important topics in general and systemic pathology. A student who is conversant with so many key facts should expect to perform well in comprehensive pathology tests, including standardized examinations.

Ivan Damjanov, M.D., Ph.D.

Emanuel Rubin, M.D.

Contents

Chapter 1

Cell Pathology

Questions

Reversible and Irreversible Cellular Changes

A. Apoptosis
B. Atrophy
C. Caseous necrosis
D. Coagulative necrosis
E. Dysplasia
F. Dystrophic calcification
G. Fat necrosis
H. Fatty change
I. Fibrinoid necrosis
J. Glycogen accumulation
K. Hemosiderin
L. Hydropic (vacuolar) change
M. Hyperplasia
N. Hypertrophy
O. Karyorrhexis
P. Liquefactive necrosis
Q. Mallory's hyalin
R. Metaplasia
S. Metastatic calcification
T. Pyknosis

_____ 1. Enlarged arm and leg muscles in an athlete

_____ 2. Programmed cell death that normally occurs in developing fetal limbs

_____ 3. Reversible cell swelling in renal tubules caused by hypoperfusion of the kidneys during open heart surgery

_____ 4. Saponification of peripancreatic tissue following an attack of acute pancreatitis

_____ 5. Softened localized area in the brain (encephalomalacia) caused by an occlusion of the middle cerebral artery

_____ 6. Yellowish-white soft area in a lymph node infected with *Mycobacterium tuberculosis*

_____ 7. Transformation of glandular endocervical epithelium into squamous epithelium in chronic cervicitis

_____ 8. Myositis ossificans is an example of this pathological process.

_____ 9. Alcohol-induced changes in the liver recognizable on gross or microscopic examination

_____ 10. Preneoplastic changes seen in the bronchial mucosa of smokers

_____ 11. Carbon tetrachloride–induced irreversible nuclear changes in the liver characterized by shrinkage of nuclei and compaction of chromatin

_____ 12. Round, anuclear, acidophilic bodies in the liver infected with hepatitis B virus

_____ 13. Small brown heart in a 90-year-old man

_____ 14. Estrogen-induced thickening of the endometrium

_____ 15. Cytoplasmic bodies composed of aggregates of cytoskeletal filaments in hepatocytes of chronic alcoholics

_____ 16. Vacuolated liver cells in frozen sections that stain positively with Sudan red or oil red O

_____ 17. Firm, pale, kidney infarct caused by occlusion of a branch of a renal artery

_____ 18. Fragmented nuclei ("nuclear dust") in an infarct of the kidney

_____ 19. Pompe disease

_____ 20. Response of thymic lymphocytes to corticosteroid treatment

_____ 21. Hardened deformed cardiac valves in a 40-year-old patient who had rheumatic endocarditis 20 years ago

_____ 22. Hardening of coronary arteries in a 60-year-old man who had diabetes for 20 years

_____ 23. Deposits of calcium phosphate crystals in kidney parenchyma of a patient who had a parathyroid adenoma

_____ 24. Partially calcified alveolar septa in the lungs of a patient with breast cancer metastatic to bone

_____ 25. Osteoporosis

_____ 26. Pigment in the dark brown liver of a patient who had hereditary hemolytic anemia

_____ 27. Type of necrosis that is found in an abscess

_____ 28. Enlargement of the heart and thickening of left ventricle due to hypertension

_____ 29. The most common cause of prostatic enlargement in aging men

_____ 30. Brown pigment that accumulates in hereditary hemochromatosis and gives a positive Prussian blue reaction

_____ 31. Histologic change in the wall of muscular arteries affected by autoimmune diseases such as polyarteritis nodosa or systemic lupus erythematosus

DIRECTIONS: Choose the one best answer.

_____ 32. Hydropic swelling of the cell is characterized by all the following *except*
A. increased number of cytoplasmic organelles.
B. dilatation of cisternae of endoplasmic reticulum.
C. impairment of cellular volume regulation.
D. influx of sodium into the cell.
E. efflux of potassium from the cell.

_____ 33. All the following are examples of atrophy *except*
A. skeletal muscle, following transection of its motor neuron.
B. skeletal muscles, following long-term immobilization of the broken extremity in a cast.
C. ovary following hypophysectomy.
D. endometrium following long-term administration of estrogen.
E. brain of a 100-year-old man.

_____ 34. Hypertrophic heart muscle cells contain increased amounts of
A. water in the sarcoplasmic reticulum.
B. smooth endoplasmic reticulum.
C. peroxisomes.
D. phagosomes.
E. messenger RNA.

_____ 35. Erythroid hyperplasia of the bone marrow is often found in people who live
A. at sea level, as in San Diego.
B. at high altitude, as in the Andes.
C. in equatorial jungles of Brazil.
D. above the polar circle in Canada.
E. around the Great Lakes, as in Chicago or Cleveland.

_____ 36. Squamous metaplasia occurs typically in
A. bronchi of chronic smokers.
B. skin exposed to sunlight.
C. a callus.
D. Barrett esophagus.
E. chronic gastritis.

_____ 37. Which of the following pathologic processes is an example of dysplasia?
A. Actinic keratosis
B. Chronic cystitis
C. Chronic bronchitis
D. Ulcerative colitis
E. Barrett esophagus

_____ 38. All the following accumulate reversibly in the liver cells *except*
A. lipid from fatty food.
B. iron from hemolyzed red blood cells.
C. carbon particles.
D. vitamin B_{12}.
E. glycogen.

_____ 39. Yellow brown granules were found in liver cells and Kupffer cells of a man with hereditary hemochromatosis. These granules became blue following the Prussian blue reaction. What are these granules?
A. Transferrin
B. Hemosiderin
C. Hemoglobin
D. Bilirubin
E. Biliverdin

_____ 40. All the following are signs of necrosis *except*
A. lipofuscin.
B. pyknosis.
C. karyolysis.
D. karyorrhexis.
E. cell membrane rupture.

_____ 41. Enzymatic necrosis affecting the pancreas is called
A. coagulative necrosis.
B. liquefactive necrosis.
C. fat necrosis.
D. caseous necrosis.
E. fibrinoid necrosis.

_____ 42. Which cation is found in extremely high concentrations in cells that have undergone coagulative necrosis?
A. Potassium
B. Calcium
C. Iron
D. Cobalt
E. Copper

_____ 43. Which of the following cell types is least sensitive to anoxia?
A. Neurons
B. Cardiac myocytes
C. Small intestinal absorptive cells
D. Proximal renal tubule cells
E. Fibroblasts

_____ 44. Reperfusion injury is characterized by the formation of potentially toxic substances that are best classified as
A. lysosomal enzymes.
B. proteases.
C. activated oxygen species.
D. hydrogen.
E. hydrochloric acid.

_____ 45. Lipid peroxidation in cells exposed to ionizing radiation is initiated by
A. catalase.
B. superoxide.
C. hydroxyl radical.
D. hydrogen peroxide.
E. glutathione.

_____ **46.** Indirectly cytopathic viruses kill cells by provoking an
A. injury to DNA.
B. injury to RNA.
C. injury to the cell membrane.
D. influx of potassium.
E. immune response.

_____ **47.** Carbon tetrachloride, acetaminophen, and bromobenzene—three well-known hepatotoxins—form reactive toxic metabolites within the liver cells after they have been metabolized in the
A. nucleus.
B. nucleolus.
C. Golgi apparatus.
D. smooth endoplasmic reticulum.
E. mitochondria.

_____ **48.** Which of the following is typical of apoptosis?
A. Activation of DNA synthesis, as in the mitotic cycle
B. Activation of endogenous endonucleases
C. Reduced cytosolic free calcium
D. Karyolysis
E. Inflammation in the tissue

_____ **49.** Which of the following represents an example of metastatic calcification?
A. Old foci of tuberculosis in the lymph nodes
B. Mitral valve damaged by rheumatic fever
C. Calcific mitral stenosis
D. Breast cancer visible by mammography
E. Pulmonary calcification in chronic renal failure

_____ **50.** Which of the following statements about aging is true?
A. Zoo animals have shorter lifespans than animals in their normal habitat.
B. All animal species have approximately the same lifespan.
C. Men are programmed to live longer than women.
D. Identical twins have a natural lifespan of approximately similar duration.
E. Fibroblasts of different species explanted in vitro have the same lifespan.

_____ **51.** All the following are typical structural changes that accompany aging *except*
A. loss of pulmonary vital capacity.
B. decreased velocity of nerve conductance.
C. increased amount of water in tissues.
D. decreased total body fat.
E. increased amount of lipofuscin in tissues.

_____ **52.** Which of the following cytoplasmic structures contains fragmented mitochondria?
A. Golgi apparatus
B. Primary lysosomes
C. Heterophagosomes
D. Autophagosomes
E. Pinocytotic vacuoles

_____**53.**   Squamous metaplasia of cigarette smokers is typically seen in the epithelium lining the
A. oral cavity.
B. epiglottis.
C. bronchi.
D. alveoli.
E. pleural surfaces.

_____ **54.** Metastatic calcification is seen in
A. vitamin A deficiency.
B. vitamin D deficiency.
C. hyperparathyroidism.
D. hypothyroidism.
E. heart failure.

_____ **55.** Increased amounts of calcium in the cytosol of an injured cell reflect a release of calcium from stores in the
A. nucleus.
B. smooth endoplasmic reticulum.
C. lysosomes.
D. mitochondria.
E. peroxisomes.

Answers

1. **The answer is N.** Exercise leads to *hypertrophy* of skeletal muscle cells. Since the skeletal muscle cells cannot divide, hyperplasia does not occur in this tissue.

2. **The answer is A.** Programmed cell death that normally occurs during the formation of many fetal parts and organs, including fetal limbs, is called *apoptosis*. In fetal limb buds, apoptosis involves the cells between the fetal fingers and toes. Without apoptosis the fingers and toes do not separate, resulting in syndactyly.

3. **The answer is L.** Reversible hypoxic cell injury leads to an influx of sodium and water into the cell and is called *hydropic or vacuolar change*. It occurs often in kidneys that do not receive enough oxygenated blood during prolonged surgical operations. If the blood flow is restored, the swollen tubular cells resume their normal shape and function, indicating that hydropic change is reversible.

4. **The answer is G.** Saponification of fat derived from peripancreatic fat cells exposed to pancreatic enzymes is a typical feature of enzymatic *fat necrosis*. Lipase, released from pancreatic acinar cells during an attack of acute pancreatitis hydrolyzes fat into fatty acids and glycerol. Fatty acids bind with calcium to form soaps—a process known as saponification. Entry of calcium ions into the injured tissue reduces the level of calcium in blood. Hypocalcemia is therefore a typical finding in patients who had a bout of acute pancreatitis.

5. **The answer is P.** Brain infarcts are typically soft and diffluent and are examples of *liquefactive necrosis*. The term *encephalomalacia*, derived from the Greek term for brain softening, is a synonym for *brain infarcts*. The

portion of the brain supplied by the middle cerebral artery is the most common site of cerebral infarcts.

6. **The answer is C.** Yellowish-white, cheesy material in a lymph node infected with *M. tuberculosis* represents an area of *caseous necrosis*. This lesion occurs in the center of many infectious granulomas, such as those evoked by *M. tuberculosis, Histoplasma capsulatum*, and many other deep fungal infections.

7. **The answer is R.** Transformation of glandular into squamous epithelium represents squamous *metaplasia*. In the endocervix it is most often a response to chronic infection.

8. **The answer is R.** Myositis ossificans is a disease characterized by formation of bony trabeculae within striated muscle. It represents a form of osseous *metaplasia*.

9. **The answer is H.** *Fatty change* of the liver is the most common lesion induced in the liver by alcohol and can be recognized on either gross or microscopic examination. On sectioning, the fatty liver is enlarged, yellow, and greasy. Microscopically, the fat-laden cells appear vacuolated in sections prepared from paraffin-embedded tissue because the fat has been extracted during processing in solvents.

10. **The answer is E.** *Dysplasia* of the bronchial epithelium is a reaction of respiratory epithelium to carcinogens in tobacco smoke. Dysplasia is reversible, if the affected person stops smoking, but it may also progress to carcinoma. Hence, it is considered preneoplastic.

11. **The answer is T.** Compaction of chromatin in dying or dead cells is called *pyknosis*. Together with karyolysis and karyorrhexis, pyknosis is one of the morphologic signs of irreversible cell injury and cell death.

12. **The answer is A.** Acidophilic, round, anuclear bodies in a liver infected with hepatitis B virus represent a form of virus-induced *apoptosis*. Acidophilic bodies were first described in another viral disease (yellow fever) and are also known as Councilman bodies.

13. **The answer is B.** A small brown heart in a nonagenarian is an example of senile *atrophy*. The brown color of the myocardium reflects the accumulation of the brown pigment lipofuscin.

14. **The answer is M.** Estrogen-induced thickening of the endometrium represents *hyperplasia*. Estrogen stimulates the proliferation of endometrial glands and stroma. If unopposed by progesterone (as normally occurs in the secretory phase of the menstrual cycle), it will cause the marked thickening of typical endometrial hyperplasia. The hyperplastic endometrium contains an increased number of both stromal and glandular cells.

15. **The answer is Q.** Cytoplasmic bodies composed of keratin-rich intermediate filaments are known as *Mallory hyalin*.

16. **The answer is H.** Vacuolization of liver cells could represent several processes: (a) hydropic change reflecting an influx of sodium and water; (b) accumulation of glycogen, as in glycogen storage diseases or diabetes; or (c) *fatty change* marked by the accumulation of triglycerides. Large fat droplets are distinctive because they occupy most of the cytoplasm, displacing the compressed ("semilunar") liver cell nucleus to the periphery. Smaller fat droplets ("microvesicular" fatty change, as seen in

Reye syndrome or tetracycline toxicity) are less distinct and can be confused with nonlipid vacuoles. To prove the lipid nature of cytoplasmic vacuoles, one must use lipophilic dyes, such as Sudan red or oil red O.

17. **The answer is D.** Typical ischemic (pale) infarcts of solid internal organs such as the kidney represent areas of *coagulative necrosis*.

18. **The answer is O.** Nuclear fragments in necrotic tissue are evidence of *karyorrhexis*.

19. **The answer is J.** Pompe disease (glycogenosis type II) is an inborn error or metabolism that leads to the *accumulation of glycogen* in the cytoplasm of the liver, heart, and skeletal muscle cells. This congenital acid maltase deficiency results in the storage of glycogen within lysosomes.

20. **The answer is A.** Corticosteroid treatment leads to *apoptosis* of thymic lymphocytes.

21. **The answer is F.** Hardening of cardiac valves after damage by rheumatic fever reflects *dystrophic calcification*.

22. **The answer is F.** Atherosclerotic coronary arteries are hardened because their walls contain large deposits of calcium salts. The serum levels of calcium are normal, and the calcium deposits are located in previously damaged tissue. Such *calcification* is called *dystrophic*.

23. **The answer is S.** Parathyroid adenomas produce large quantities of parathyroid hormone, which leads to hypercalcemia. *Calcification* of renal parenchyma in the presence of hypercalcemia termed *metastatic*.

24. **The answer is S.** Breast cancer metastases to bone are often osteolytic and accompanied by hypercalcemia. Excess calcium gives rise to *metastatic calcification* of normal tissues.

25. **The answer is B.** Osteoporosis represents an *atrophy* of bony trabeculae and cortical bone. Such bones are brittle and prone to fracture.

26. **The answer is K.** In hemolytic anemia the liver becomes dark brown because of *hemosiderin,* which accumulates primarily in Kupffer cells and to a lesser extent in hepatocytes. Hemosiderin is an iron-containing pigment derived from the hemoglobin of hemolyzed red blood cells.

27. **The answer is P.** Abscess, a cavity filled with pus, represents a form of *liquefactive necrosis*. Lytic enzymes released from dead and dying leukocytes lead to the liquefaction of tissue.

28. **The answer is N.** Heart responds to increased demand posed by hypertension by undergoing *hypertrophy*. Since the cardiac myocytes cannot divide, hyperplasia cannot take place in the heart.

29. **The answer is M.** Hormonally induced *hyperplasia* is the most common cause of prostatic enlargement in aging men.

30. **The answer is K.** Patients affected by hereditary hemochromatosis cannot regulate the uptake of iron in the small intestine. Excess iron accumulates initially as *hemosiderin* in normal storage sites (bone marrow, spleen, liver). However, once the storage capacity of these organs is exceeded, hemosiderin deposits are found in other organs as well. Hemosiderin granules are brown and form a blue pigment when exposed to ferri-ferrocyanide (Prussian blue reaction). This histochemi-

cal Prussian blue reaction is used to distinguish hemosiderin from other brown pigments (e.g., bile, melanin, or lipofuscin).

31. **The answer is I.** Arteries affected by polyarteritis nodosa or systemic lupus erythematosus (SLE) show signs of *fibrinoid necrosis.*

32. **The answer is A.** Except for A, all the answers describe changes that typically occur during hydropic swelling. The volume of the cell increases because of an influx of sodium and water into the cytoplasm. *The number of cytoplasmic organelles remains the same.*

33. **The answer is D.** All answers except for D are examples of atrophy. Atrophy of skeletal muscles can result from a loss of innervation due to spinal cord or peripheral nerve trauma. Inactivity, as is often seen following the long-term immobilization of an extremity in a cast, has the same effect. Hypophysectomy is accompanied by atrophy of the thyroid, adrenal cortex, and ovary, which are all organs that depend on stimulation by pituitary trophic hormones. The brain atrophies with advancing age. *Estrogen exerts trophic effects on the endometrium, causing hyperplasia rather than atrophy.* Endometrial atrophy occurs following ovariectomy or after the menopause, when the ovaries no longer produce estrogen.

34. **The answer is E.** Hypertrophic cardiac myocytes, which are larger than normal, have more cytoplasm and larger nuclei than normal cells. The enlarged nuclei contain more DNA and RNA than their normal counterparts and generate *more messenger RNA.* The cytoplasm of hypertrophic myocytes contains more myofilaments and mitochondria, but the number of other cytoplasmic organelles is not increased. Water influx, which is typical of hydropic swelling, is not found in hypertrophy.

35. **The answer is B.** Erythroid hyperplasia is typically found in people *living at high altitude,* because low oxygen tension evokes the production of erythropoietin, which promotes the proliferation of erythroid precursors in the bone marrow.

36. **The answer is A.** Long-term smoking irritates the normal columnar *bronchial epithelium,* which undergoes squamous metaplasia (i.e., it transforms into stratified squamous epithelium). Skin cannot undergo squamous metaplasia, because it is already lined by stratified squamous epithelium. The term callus refers to thickening of the skin (e.g., as would be caused by ill-fitting shoes); it is an example of hyperplasia rather than metaplasia. Barrett's esophagus represents a form of glandular metaplasia in which the normal squamous epithelium of the esophagus changes into gastric or intestinal epithelium. In chronic gastritis the normal gastric mucosa changes into intestinal epithelium but is not converted into squamous epithelium.

37. **The answer is A.** *Actinic keratosis* is a form of dysplasia in sun-exposed skin. Histologically, such lesions are composed of atypical squamous cells, which vary in size and shape. They show no signs of regular maturation as the cells move from the basal layer of the epidermis to its surface. Dysplastic epidermis shares many features with squamous cell carcinoma, and untreated actinic keratosis often gives rise to invasive cancer. Chronic cystitis and bronchitis may result in foci of metaplasia, but these tend to be composed of differentiated cells that show no nuclear atypia. Squamous metaplasia of the columnar epithelium of the bronchi or the transitional epithelium of the urinary bladder may become dysplastic, but this transition is unpredictable. Therefore, these

metaplastic lesions should not be grouped together with actinic kerato-sis, which is often referred to as "squamous cell carcinoma, one half." Although dysplasia and even neoplasia can occur in the colonic mucosa affected by ulcerative colitis or in the columnar epithelium of Barrett's esophagus, by itself neither ulcerative colitis nor Barrett's esophagus should be classified as dysplasia.

38. **The answer is C.** Normal hepatocytes may store *lipids, iron, vitamin B₁₂,* and *glycogen* but do not store inhaled carbon particles. Carbon particles inhaled into the lungs are taken up by macrophages, which carry these particles into the hilar lymph nodes.

39. **The answer is B.** In hereditary hemochromatosis, a genetic abnormality of iron absorption in the small intestine, excess iron is stored mostly in the form of *hemosiderin,* primarily in the liver, but also in many other organs. Hemosiderin appears as brown cytoplasmic granules, which turn blue with the Prussian blue reaction. Transferrin is the plasma pro-tein that transports iron. Hemoglobin is the red iron-containing pigment of red blood cells. Upon hemolysis of red blood cells, hemoglobin is degraded into greenish biliverdin or yellow bilirubin. Bilirubin may accumulate in the liver cells, but it does not form granules that are Pruss-ian-blue positive.

40. **The answer is A.** Lipofuscin, also known as "wear and tear pigment," appears in the form of brown granules in the cytoplasm of living cells but is not a sign of necrosis. *Pyknosis, karyolysis,* and *karyorrhexis* are terms that describe nuclear changes in dead or irreversibly injured cells. *Cell membrane rupture* is also associated with cell death, and is a sign of irreversible cell injury.

41. **The answer is C.** Enzyme-mediated necrosis of pancreas and peripan-creatic fat tissue is called *fat necrosis*. Release of lipolytic enzymes from the injured pancreas leads to enzymatic degradation of triglycerides into glycerol and fatty acids, which combine with calcium and are deposited at the site of necrosis as calcium soaps.

42. **The answer is B.** Coagulative necrosis is characterized by a massive influx of *calcium* into the cell. Under normal circumstances the plasma membrane maintains a steep gradient of calcium ions, whose concentra-tion in interstitial fluids is 10,000 times higher than that inside the cell. Irreversible cell injury damages the plasma membrane, which then fails to maintain this gradient, thereby allowing the influx of calcium into the cell.

43. **The answer is E.** Highly specialized cells, such as neurons, cardiac myocytes, small intestinal absorptive cells, and cells of the proximal renal tubule, are much more sensitive to anoxia than are *fibroblasts*. The former require more oxygen for maintenance of their complex functions.

44. **The answer is C.** Toxic *activated oxygen species* are formed in tissues dur-ing the reperfusion of an infarcted area. Oxygen radicals are formed inside the cells through the xanthine oxidase pathway but are also released from neutrophils that have entered the infarcted area.

45. **The answer is C.** Radiolysis of water leads to formation of *hydroxyl rad-icals* that initiate lipid peroxidation of membrane phospholipids.

46. **The answer is E.** In contrast to directly cytopathic viruses, which cause cell death by damaging the cell membrane indirectly, cytopathic viruses

produce antigenic proteins that are inserted into the cell membrane and are capable of evoking an *immune response.* Attack by immune lymphocytes, which recognize the viral protein as foreign, destroys the cell membrane.

47. **The answer is D.** Most chemicals, including the three hepatotoxins listed here, are metabolized in the *smooth endoplasmic reticulum* by mixed function oxidases, which convert these chemicals into highly reactive radicals. For example, addition of an electron to CCl_4 results in the formation of a trichloramethyl radical, which damages the cell membrane by initiating lipoperoxidation. Reactive lipid radicals diffuse from the endoplasmic reticulum into other parts of the cell, ultimately damaging the plasma membrane and causing cell death.

48. **The answer is B.** Apoptosis is characterized by the activation of *endonucleases,* which leads to DNA fragmentation. The chromatin of apoptotic nuclei appears clumped as in pyknosism, but karolysis does not occur. Nuclei may become fragmented, but this fragmentation is distinct from mitotic division. Apoptosis does not induce an influx of inflammatory cells, and the dead cell fragments are taken up by adjacent cells in the tissue itself. Similar to other forms of cell death, apoptosis is associated with an influx of calcium into the cytosol.

49. **The answer is E.** *End-stage renal failure* leads to hyperparathyroidism and secondarily to hypercalcemia. The latter results in metastatic calcification. Old foci of tuberculosis, a calcified mitral valve damaged previously by rheumatic fever, and calcification within breast cancer are all examples of *dystrophic* calcification.

50. **The answer is D.** *Identical twins* have a life span of approximately the same duration, which supports a genetic influence on aging. Life in the protected environment does not prolong life: animals in zoos tend to live longer than those in the wild. Different species vary with regard to their lifespans. The same holds true for their fibroblasts explanted in vitro. A greater female longevity is almost universal in the animal kingdom, but the reasons are not known.

51. **The answer is D.** Aging is accompanied by *increased* rather than decreased total *body fat.* The tissues contain more lipofuscin, the "wear and tear" pigment. With aging there is progressive decrease in many vital functions, including pulmonary vital capacity, velocity of nerve conductance, cardiac contractility, and glomerular filtration.

52. **The answer is D.** *Autophagosomes* are lysosome derived phagocytic vacuoles filled with fragments of old or damaged organelles.

53. **The answer is C.** Cigarette smoking leads to squamous metaplasia of the columnar epithelium lining the *bronchi.*

54. **The answer is C.** *Hyperparathyroidism* causes hypercalcemia, a prerequisite for metastatic calcification.

55. **The answer is D.** Increased amounts of calcium in the cytosol of an injured cell result from an influx from extracellular space, mitochondria, and rough endoplasmic reticulum.

Chapter 2

Inflammation

Questions

DIRECTIONS: Match each numbered statement with the most appropriate lettered item. Each lettered item can be used once, more than once, or not at all.

Mediators of Inflammation

A. Arachidonic acid
B. Bradykinin
C. Complement system
D. Cytokines
E. Defensin
F. Hageman factor
G. Histamine
H. Integrins
I. Kallikrein
J. Leukotrienes
K. Lipocortin
L. Membrane attack complex
M. Nitric oxide
N. Opsonin
O. Platelet activating factor (PAF)
P. Prostacyclin (PGI_2)
Q. Prostaglandin E_2
R. Selectin
S. Thromboxane A_2
T. Tumor necrosis factor

_____ **1.** Corticosteroid-induced inhibitor of phospholipase A_2, which blocks the formation of arachidonic acid from phosphatidylcholine

_____ **2.** Arachidonic acid derivative produced in the cyclooxygenase pathway that causes vasoconstriction and bronchoconstriction

_____ **3.** Arachidonic acid derivative produced in the cyclooxygenase pathway that causes vasodilatation and bronchodilatation

_____ 4. Endothelial cell–derived low-molecular-weight vasodilator that also inhibits platelet aggregation

_____ 5 Biogenic amine released from mast cells after exposure to cold

_____ 6. Arachidonic acid derivatives that mediate asthma

_____ 7. Edema-promoting substance released from mast cells exposed to C3a and C5a components of complement

_____ 8. Vasoactive acetylated lysophospholipid generated upon stimulation of all inflammatory cells. It primes phagocytic cells to form more oxygen radicals upon exposure to a second stimulus.

_____ 9. This enzyme generated by the action of activated Hageman factor cleaves high-molecular-weight kininogen to produce bradykinin and acts autocatalytically to produce more activated Hageman factor.

_____ 10. The precursor of prostaglandins that is formed from membrane phospholipids through the action of phospholipase A2

_____ 11. Serum factor that activates the complement cascade and the coagulation and fibrinolytic systems

_____ 12. Lipid-soluble cytolytic protein complex formed by the activation of complement system

_____ 13. Polypeptides that induce secretion of acute response reactants in the liver

_____ 14. Substances that facilitate phagocytosis of bacteria

_____ 15. Glycoproteins stored in Weibel-Palade bodies and redistributed in early stages of inflammation on endothelial cell surfaces. They mediate loose adhesion of leukocytes and their rolling along the endothelial surfaces.

_____ 16. Cationic bactericidal proteins released from primary granules of polymorphonuclear leukocytes

_____ 17. Polypeptide factors produced by activated lymphocytes and macrophages, which are involved in endothelial cell activation

_____ 18. Arachidonic acid derivative induced in the hypothalamic thermoregulatory centers by TNF and IL-1

_____ 19. Cell adhesion molecules, belonging to the immunoglobulin family, expressed on both endothelial cells and leukocytes. They mediate leukocyte endothelial cell firm adhesion and transmigration of leukocytes across the vascular wall.

_____ 20. A group of proteins that is activated in a cascade. They form biologically active fragments and complexes that increase vascular permeability and have chemotactic, cytolytic, and opsonic functions.

Morphologic Features and Signs of Inflammation

A. Abscess
B. Acute phase reactants
C. Callus
D. Empyema
E. Eosinophilia
F. Fibrinous inflammation

G. Fibrosis
H. Fistula
I. Gangrene
J. Granulation tissue
K. Granuloma, caseating
L. Granuloma, noncaseating
M. Keloid
N. Leukocytosis
O. Leukopenia
P. Lymphocytosis
Q. Lymphopenia
R. Pyosalpinx
S. Septicemia
T. Serous inflammation

_____ **21.** A patient known to have endocarditis presents with shaking chills, bacteriologically positive blood cultures, and a brain abscess. Which diagnosis encompasses all these findings?

_____ **22.** Four weeks after a complex fracture of the femur the bone defect contained fibrous tissue and newly formed irregular bone spicules. What is the term used for the tissue that replaces the normal bone at the fracture site?

_____ **23.** It is typically found on peripheral blood examination in infectious mononucleosis.

_____ **24.** Typical tissue and peripheral blood finding in patients infected with *Trichinella spiralis*

_____ **25.** Typical peripheral blood finding in acute appendicitis

_____ **26.** Typical peripheral blood finding in typhoid fever and some rickettsial diseases

_____ **27.** These proteins are synthesized by liver cells stimulated with cytokines, such as IL-6, and account to some extent for an increased erythrocyte sedimentation rate in inflammatory diseases.

_____ **28.** Hypertrophic scar

_____ **29.** Blister caused by heat

_____ **30.** Rheumatic pericarditis, characterized by a shaggy white exudate loosely adherent to the epicardium and pericardium, and commonly described at autopsy as "bread and butter" type exudate.

_____ **31.** Typically found in tuberculous lymphadenitis

_____ **32.** The name for dense collagenous adhesions between epicardium and pericardium, typical of constrictive pericarditis

_____ **33.** An encapsulated localized collection of pus within the brain tissue

_____ **34.** Necrotic, infected foot of a diabetic

_____ **35.** Collection of pus in the pleural cavity complicating staphylococcal pneumonia

_____ **36.** Accumulation of pus in the fallopian tubes, typical of pelvic inflammatory disease (PID)

_____ **37.** A probe-patent tract connecting vagina and rectum

_____ **38.** Typical pathologic lesion of sarcoidosis

_____ **39.** Tissue composed of fibroblasts, angioblasts, and macrophages filling the bottom of a surgical wound 5 days after operation

_____ **40.** Peripheral blood count finding in endotoxemia

_____ **41.** Peripheral blood count finding in AIDS

DIRECTIONS: Choose the one best answer.

_____ **42.** The initial reaction to neurogenic and chemical stimuli in an area of inflammation is a transient
A. dilatation of arterioles.
B. constriction of arterioles.
C. constriction of venules.
D. dilatation of venules.
E. constriction of capillaries.

_____ **43.** Endothelial cells that react most prominently to mediators of inflammation are found in the
A. muscular arteries.
B. elastic arteries.
C. arterioles.
D. venules.
E. veins.

_____ **44.** Which of the following statements about exudate and transudate is true?
A. A transudate results from rupture of the vessel wall in a noninflammatory process.
B. An exudate contains more protein than transudate.
C. A transudate contains more cells than exudate.
D. A transudate is usually purulent.
E. A transudate contains a great deal of cellular debris.

_____ **45.** All the following statements about vasoactive mediators of inflammation are true *except*
A. they may be derived from inflammatory cells.
B. they may be derived from plasma.
C. they may be derived from vascular smooth muscle cells.
D. in plasma they are usually inactive unless activated at the site of inflammation.
E. their action is usually counterbalanced by that of natural inhibitors.

_____ **46.** Slow-reacting substances of anaphylaxis are derived from
A. arachidonic acid through the cyclooxygenase pathway.
B. arachidonic acid through the lipoxygenase pathway.
C. alternate complement pathway.
D. classical complement pathway.
E. histones.

_____ 47. Which of the following preformed substances released from mast cells and platelets increases the permeability of blood vessels?

A. Leukotriene
B. Phospholipase
C. Histamine
D. Bradykinin
E. Hageman factor

_____ 48. Platelet activating factor (PAF) has all the following actions *except*

A. promotes aggregation of platelets.
B. promotes degranulation of platelets.
C. stimulates the release of vasoactive substances from platelets.
D. stimulates the motility of leukocytes.
E. causes vasoconstriction of arterioles.

_____ 49. The activation of Hageman factor causes all the following *except*

A. clotting.
B. fibrinolysis.
C. complement activation.
D. kinin generation.
E. reverse transcriptase activation.

_____ 50. Bradykinin is a vasoactive polypeptide of low molecular weight formed from a high-molecular-weight precursor (kininogen) in the plasma. This occurs through the action of an enzyme known as

A. tryptase.
B. alpha-1-antitrypsin.
C. plasminogen activator.
D. kallikrein.
E. zymosan.

_____ 51. The membrane attack complex formed by the complement cascade is

A. lipid insoluble.
B. capable of lysing cells.
C. a complement fragment.
D. formed only in the classical complement pathway.
E. formed through the action of bradykinin.

_____ 52. Complement-derived anaphylatoxins such as C3a and C5a have all the following effects *except*

A. bronchoconstriction.
B. vasoconstriction.
C. increased vascular permeability.
D. chemotaxis.
E. fibrinolysis.

_____ 53. The process by which complement fragments and complexes coat bacteria and enhance phagocytosis by leukocytes is called
   A. margination.
   B. pavementing.
   C. chemotaxis.
   D. opsonization.
   E. aggregation.

_____ 54. Which chemotactic factor acting on leukocytes is formed from bacteria and mitochondrial membranes?
   A. HPETE
   B. Leukotriene B4
   C. N-formylated peptide
   D. bradykinin
   E. Hageman factor

_____ 55. Which of the following substances is found only in the primary granules of neutrophils and not in other granules?
   A. Acid hydrolases
   B. Alkaline phosphatase
   C. Cationic proteins
   D. Lysozyme
   E. Histamine

_____ 56. Myeloperoxidase is found in
   A. neutrophils.
   B. macrophages.
   C. epithelioid cells.
   D. basophils.
   E. lymphocytes.

_____ 57. Which of the following plasma proteins inhibits plasmin-activated fibrinolysis and the activation of the complement system?
   A. Alkaline phosphatase
   B. Acid phosphatase
   C. Myeloperoxidase
   D. α_2-Macroglobulin
   E. Lactoferrin

_____ 58. A localized purulent infection contained within the parenchyma of an organ is called
   A. empyema.
   B. sinus.
   C. fistula.
   D. abscess.
   E. phlegmon.

_____ 59. The principal cells of granulomatous inflammation are
   A. lymphocytes and plasma cells.
   B. plasma cells and macrophages.
   C. macrophages and lymphocytes.
   D. giant cells and plasma cells.
   E. giant cells and neutrophils.

_____ **60.** Foreign-body giant cells are derived from
   A. lymphocytes.
   B. macrophages.
   C. basophils.
   D. eosinophils.
   E. mast cells.

_____ **61.** Parasitic infestations typically provoke
   A. leukopenia.
   B. neutrophilia.
   C. eosinophilia.
   D. lymphocytosis.
   E. lymphopenia.

_____ **62.** A high white cell count in an acute viral infection is marked by an increased number of
   A. neutrophils.
   B. basophils.
   C. eosinophils.
   D. lymphocytes.
   E. plasma cells.

_____ **63.** The main endogenous pyrogen in humans is
   A. arachidonic acid.
   B. leukotriene B4.
   C. interleukin-1.
   D. prostacyclin.
   E. thromboxane.

_____ **64.** Caseating granulomas are typical of a reaction to
   A. viruses.
   B. *Mycobacterium tuberculosis*.
   C. parasites.
   D. pyogenic bacteria.
   E. foreign bodies.

Answers

1. **The answer is K.** *Lipocortin* is a corticosteroid-induced inhibitor of phospholipase A_2. It mediates the anti-inflammatory effects of corticosteroids.

2. **The answer is S.** *Thromboxane A_2*, a derivative of arachidonic acid formed in the cyclooxygenase pathway, promotes vasoconstriction, bronchoconstriction, and platelet aggregation.

3. **The answer is P.** *Prostacyclin*, a derivative of arachidonic acid, is formed in the cyclooxygenase pathway. It promotes vasodilatation and bronchodilatation but inhibits platelet aggregation. Its action is diametrically opposite to that of thromboxane A_2.

4. **The answer is M.** *Nitric oxide* (NO), previously known as endothelium-derived relaxing factor (EDRF), leads to relaxation of vascular smooth muscle cells and vasodilatation of arterioles. NO also inhibits platelet

aggregation and mediates the killing of bacteria and tumor cells by macrophages.

5. **The answer is G.** *Histamine*, a biogenic amine stored in cytoplasmic granules of mast cells, is released in response to a variety of stimuli, including cold or heat, mechanical pressure, and various chemicals. In type I hypersensitivity reactions, histamine release is triggered by an antigen/antibody reaction, which takes place on the surface of IgE-coated mast cells.

6. **The answer is J.** *Leukotrienes*, also known as slow-reacting substances of anaphylaxis (SRS-As), are potent bronchoconstrictors and are the main mediators of asthma. Leukotrienes are formed from arachidonic acid through the lipoxygenase pathway.

7. **The answer is G.** *Histamine* released from mast cells exposed to C3a and C5a causes increased vascular permeability and localized edema. Massive release of histamine may cause anaphylactic shock. Hence, C3a and C5a are termed *anaphylatoxins*.

8. **The answer is O.** *Platelet-activating factor (PAF)* is a multifactorial lysophospholipid produced by most, if not all, cells that are activated in inflammation. PAF induces platelet aggregation and degranulation, augments arachidonic acid metabolism, and primes leukocytes to form more oxygen radicals.

9. **The answer is I.** *Kallikrein* is an enzyme formed from prekallikrein that is exposed to activated Hageman factor. It generates bradykinin from high-molecular-weight kininogen (HMWK). Once formed, kallikrein acts autocatalytically, producing more activated Hageman factor, which in turn converts more prekallikrein into kallikrein.

10. **The answer is A.** *Arachidonic acid* is formed from membrane phospholipids through the action of phospholipase A_2. Arachidonic acid is metabolized through two pathways—the lipoxygenase and the cyclooxygenase pathways. Prostaglandins are formed though the cyclooxygenase pathway.

11. **The answer is F.** *Hageman factor* is a pivotal serum protein that activates complement, kinin, coagulation, and the fibrinolytic system.

12. **The answer is L.** The *membrane attack complex* (MAC) is formed from terminal polypeptides of the complement cascade (C5b-C9) and inserts into the cell membranes of erythrocytes and other cells, causing their lysis.

13. **The answer is D.** *Cytokines* such as interleukins (IL-1, IL-2, etc.) are polypeptides produced by activated lymphocytes, macrophages, and many other cells. Among numerous functions, they stimulate the liver to produce acute phase reactants (e.g., C-reactive protein, transferrin, ceruloplasmin, serum amyloid-A precursor protein, and others).

14. **The answer is N.** *Opsonin* is the collective name for substances that facilitate the phagocytosis of bacteria. The most important opsonins are fragments and intermediate complexes formed in the activated complement cascade and immunoglobulin G (IgG).

15. **The answer is R.** *Selectins* are adhesive glycoproteins that mediate the initial loose adhesion of leukocytes to endothelial cells in inflammation. E selectins are found on endothelial cells, P selectins on platelets, and L selectins on leukocytes. E selectins are stored in Weibel-Palade bodies of

resting endothelial cells. Upon endothelial cell activation, E selectins are redistributed along the luminal surface of the endothelial cells, where they mediate the initial loose adhesion and rolling of leukocytes.

16. **The answer is E.** *Defensins* are bactericidal cationic proteins released from primary granules (lysosomes) of polymorphonuclear leukocytes. They increase vascular permeability and promote chemotaxis.

17. **The answer is D.** *Cytokines* mediate endothelial cell activation by causing increased synthesis and secretion of thromboxane A_2, PAF, other cytokines, and redistribution of selectins and integrins along the luminal cell surface.

18. **The answer is Q.** *Prostaglandin E_2* (PGE$_2$) is induced in the hypothalamic thermoregulatory center by IL-1 and TNF and is considered to cause fever by raising the body thermostat. Inhibition of PGE$_2$ synthesis by aspirin lowers the raised body temperature.

19. **The answer is H.** *Integrins* such as ICAM-1 or VCAM-1 are adhesion molecules that mediate the adhesion of leukocytes to endothelial cells and the transmigration of leukocytes. Integrins belong to the superfamily of immunoglobin-like proteins.

20. **The answer is C.** *Complement system* activation, which may occur through the so-called classic or alternative pathway, occurs as a cascade. Complement proteins act upon one another, generating biologically active fragments (e.g., C5a, C3b) or complexes (e.g., C567). These biologically active products of complement activation cause edema by increasing the permeability of blood vessels, promote chemotaxis of leukocytes, lyse cells, and act as opsonins by coating bacteria.

21. **The answer is S.** *Septicemia*, a term synonymous with *bacteremia*, denotes the clinical condition in which bacteria are found in the circulation. Bacteremia can be suspected clinically, but the final diagnosis is made by culturing the organisms from blood. Infected vegetations on cardiac valves in bacterial endocarditis are well-known causes of bacteremia.

22. **The answer is C.** *Callus* represents a modified granulation tissue that connects the fragments of broken bone. Similar to any other granulation tissue in a healing wound, callus is initially highly vascular. As the healing proceeds, the callus becomes more fibrotic, and spicules of bone form within it. These spicules mature into lamellar bone, which undergoes restructuring and becomes indistinguishable from the preexisting bone destroyed by fracture.

23. **The answer is P.** Similar to other viral infections, infectious mononucleosis, caused by Epstein-Barr virus, is accompanied by *lymphocytosis* (i.e., an increased number of lymphocytes in peripheral blood).

24. **The answer is E.** Infections with parasites such as Trichinella are accompanied by *eosinophilia* (i.e., an increase in circulating eosinophils). Skeletal muscle, the typical site of infection, is also infiltrated by eosinophils.

25. **The answer is N.** Acute appendicitis, similar to most other bacterial infections, is accompanied by *leukocytosis*. These leukocytes tend to be segmented (polymorphonuclear) neutrophils.

26. **The answer is O.** For unknown reasons, typhoid fever and rickettsial diseases cause *leukopenia*.

27. **The answer is B.** *Acute phase reactants* are serum proteins released from the liver in response to infection. Among others, these include C-reactive protein, ceruloplasmin, transferrin, and fibrinogen. Increased plasma concentration of these proteins, combined with a decreased concentration of albumin, accounts in part for an increased erythrocyte sedimentation rate.

28. **The answer is M.** *Keloids* are hypertrophic scars that occasionally develop after surgery, burns, or trauma in susceptible persons. Keloids are more common in blacks.

29. **The answer is T.** Blister is an example of *serous inflammation*. The clear fluid filling the blister cavity represents a transudate of plasma.

30. **The answer is F.** Rheumatic pericarditis is a typical example of *fibrinous inflammation*. The exudate that causes the adherence of epicardium to the pericardium consists predominantly of fibrin. The pericardium can be peeled off the epicardium, after which the two opposing surfaces of the pericardial cavity resemble a bread-and-butter sandwich separated in two.

31. **The answer is K.** Lymph node infection with *M. tuberculosis* evokes the formation of granulomas that typically undergo central *caseous necrosis*.

32. **The answer is G.** Dense collagenous adhesions between the epicardium and pericardium represent *fibrosis*, which develops at the site of an infectious pericarditis. The exudate in the pericardial cavity becomes organized by an ingrowth of granulation tissue, which gradually transforms into a fibrotic scar that encases the heart and prevents it from expanding during diastole (constrictive pericarditis).

33. **The answer is A.** A localized, encapsulated collection of pus within an organ is called an *abscess*.

34. **The answer is I.** Infected necrotic tissue of the leg is called wet *gangrene*. Foot gangrene occurs most often in diabetics who have atherosclerosis and diabetic microangiopathy and suffer from ischemia of the extremities.

35. **The answer is D.** *Empyema* represents a collection of pus in the pleural cavity. It is most often a complication of pneumonia caused by pyogenic bacteria (e.g., such as *Staphylococcus aureus*).

36. **The answer is R.** *Pyosalpinx* represents an accumulation of pus in the fallopian tubes. It is a constant feature of pelvic inflammatory disease (PID), which may also include formation of tubo-ovarian abscesses, endometritis, and pelvic peritonitis.

37. **The answer is H.** A *fistula* is an abnormal passage that develops between the lumen of two hollow organs. Purulent inflammation dissects a path through the wall of two adjacent organs. Rectovaginal fistula, which allows feces to enter the vagina from the rectum, is a complication of transmural infections or chronic inflammation, such as Crohn disease.

38. **The answer is L.** Sarcoidosis, a disease of unknown origin, is characterized by the formation of *noncaseating granulomas*. These granulomas are sterile (i.e., they do not contain bacteria or fungi). Similar granulomas also occur in type IV (cell-mediated) hypersensitivity reactions. Sarcoidosis is therefore considered a probable autoimmune disorder.

39. **The answer is J.** *Granulation tissue* represents a temporary tissue formed during wound healing. It consists of angioblasts that form new blood vessels, fibroblasts that lay down the collagenous matrix, and macrophages that remove damaged and dead tissue. Macrophages also secrete cytokines that modulate the repair reaction.

40. **The answer is O.** Endotoxin acts on endothelial cells and promotes the adhesion of leukocytes. Pooling of leukocytes in peripheral small blood vessels causes a spurious *leukopenia*.

41. **The answer is Q.** Patients with AIDS develop *lymphopenia* because HIV is lymphocytotropic and selectively destroys CD4 (helper) T-lymphocytes.

42. **The answer is B.** The initial response of arterioles to neurogenic and chemical stimuli is transient vasoconstriction. However, shortly thereafter, vasodilatation occurs, with an increase in blood flow to the inflamed area.

43. **The answer is D.** Endothelial cells that react prominently to mediators of inflammation are found in the *venules*. This reaction leads to gap formation and increased permeability of the venules.

44. **The answer is B.** An "exudate" contains *inflammatory cells*, necrotic debris, and *serum proteins*. By contrast, a "transudate" is not inflammatory, but is rather due to leakage of fluid into the interstitial space.

45. **The answer is C.** Vasoactive mediators are derived either from plasma or from inflammatory and endothelial cells but not from smooth muscle cells.

46. **The answer is B.** Mediators of inflammation and vasoactive substances are produced from *arachidonic acid* through either the cyclooxygenase or the lipoxygenase pathway. Leukotrienes C4, D4, and E4, which are known as slow-reacting substances of anaphylaxis (SRS-As), are synthesized through the lipoxygenase pathway. The cyclooxygenase pathway results in the formation of prostaglandins and thromboxanes.

47. **The answer is C.** *Histamine* released from granules in mast cells and platelets increases vascular permeability by inducing reversible endothelial cell contraction and gap formation.

48. **The answer is E.** Platelet-activating factor (PAF) acts not only on *platelets*, but also on leukocytes and the *microvasculature*, where it causes vasodilatation and enhanced vascular permeability.

    The effects of PAF include the following:

    A. platelets
       (1) aggregation
       (2) degranulation
       (3) release of serotonin and histamine

    B. polymorphonuclear leukocytes
       (1) stimulation of motility of leukocytes
       (2) superoxide production
       (3) degranulation

    C. Blood vessels
       (1) vasodilatation
       (2) increased permeability

49. The answer is E. The activation of Hageman factor causes *clotting* by activating the coagulation system, but it can also lead to dissolution of the clot through plasmin-mediated *fibrinolysis*. The outcome of Hageman factor activation varies, depending on the balance between these pathways. It can also *activate complement* and generate *kinins*, but it is not involved in reverse transcriptase activation.

50. The answer is D. Bradykinin is a vasoactive peptide of low molecular weight, which is referred to as "kinin" rather than "anaphylatoxin." It is generated by the action of *kallikrein*, which cleaves the high-molecular-weight kininogens in the plasma. By contrast, anaphylatoxins result from the activation of Hageman factor. These are formed from complement proteins C3 and C5 in a sequence in which activated Hageman factor acts on plasminogen to form plasmin.

51. The answer is B. Activation of the complement cascade by the classical or alternative pathway leads to the cleavage of complement fragments and the formation of active enzymatic complexes. The C5b fragment aggregates with complement proteins C6, C7, C8, and C9, resulting in the polymerization of the final product, known as the "membrane-attack complex" (MAC). MAC *lyses cells* by inserting into the plasma membrane and destroying the permeability barrier.

52. The answer is B. Complement-derived anaphylatoxins cause *bronchoconstriction* and increased *vascular permeability*, and stimulate *chemotaxis* and plasminogen-mediated *fibrinolysis*. They cause *vasodilatation* rather than vasoconstriction.

53. The answer is D. The *opsonization* of bacteria, a process that facilitates and enhances their uptake and recognition by leukocytes, can be accomplished by two normal components of body fluids, namely, IgG and complement.

54. The answer is C. *N-formylated peptides* are formed from proteins in bacterial and mitochondrial membranes. The most potent chemotactic substances are (1) the C5a fragment of complement; (2) N-formylated peptides; and (3) leukotriene B4, formed from arachidonic acid through the lipoxygenase pathway.

55. The answer is A. The primary granules in neutrophils are *lysosomes*; therefore, they are rich in *acid hydrolases*, such as acid phosphatase. However, they contain other bioactive substances and enzymes. Among the bactericidal molecules, the most important are cationic proteins, phospholipase A2, and lysozyme. These bactericidal proteins are also found in the secondary granules. The latter are, however, not lysosomes and therefore do not contain acid hydrolases.

56. The answer is A. Myeloperoxidase, an important bactericidal enzyme in the primary granules of *neutrophils*, is also present in the granules of circulating monocytes. It is, however, not found in macrophages or epithelioid cells, although these are direct descendants of blood monocytes.

57. The answer is D. α_2-*Macroglobulin* is an inhibitor of several proteases that are normally found in the plasma, released from inflammatory cells, or generated in the tissues during inflammation. Thus, among other effects, α_2-macroglobulin inhibits plasmin-activated fibrinolysis and the activation of the complement system.

58. **The answer is D.** An *"abscess"* is defined as a localized purulent inflammation. It may be acute or chronic. Chronic abscesses are composed of a central cavity filled with pus, surrounded by a layer of granulation tissue or a fibrous capsule. Plasma cells are not found in granulation tissue, unless it is chronically infected or the infection is superimposed on a B cell–mediated immunologic injury. Plasma cells are found in the granulomas of syphilis, called "gummas."

59. **The answer is C.** All granulomas contain *lymphocytes* and *macrophages*.

60. **The answer is B.** Giant cells are derived from *macrophages*.

61. **The answer is C.** Parasitic infections often elicit an *eosinophilic response*, although these cells occur in many other forms of inflammation, especially IgE-mediated allergic reactions, such as hay fever and asthma.

62. **The answer is D.** Viral infections typically cause *lymphocytosis*.

63. **The answer is C.** Fever is mediated by *interleukin-1*, a low-molecular-weight protein released from macrophages.

64. **The answer is B.** Caseating granulomas are found in tuberculosis. Other infectious granulomas, especially those caused by fungi, also show central caseous necrosis. Foreign-body granulomas do not contain such foci.

Chapter 3

Healing and Repair

Questions

DIRECTIONS: Match each numbered statement with the most appropriate lettered item. Each lettered item can be used once, more than once, or not at all.

Components and Aspects of Healing and Repair

A. Angiogenesis
B. Collagen type I
C. Collagen type II
D. Collagen type III
E. Collagen type IV
F. Contracture
G. Elastic fibers
H. Epidermal growth factor
I. Fibronectin
J. Granulation tissue
K. Integrins
L. Keloid
M. Laminin
N. Myofibroblast
O. Platelet derived growth factor
P. Proteoglycans
Q. Regeneration
R. Tenascin
S. Transforming growth factor—beta
T. Wound dehiscence

_____ 1. This collagen is typically found in cartilage, vitreous humor, and nucleus pulposus.

_____ 2. This collagen is a major component of subcutis, bones, and tendons; it is composed of repeating triplet sequences of amino acids (Gly-X-Y) and is rich in hydroxyproline and hydroxylysine.

_____ 3. Triple helix of chains of this hydroxyproline-rich basement membrane protein are interrupted by globular domains.

_____ 4. This cross-like glycoprotein of basement membranes mediates cell adhesion to basement membranes.

_____ 5. This triple helix molecule, resistant to nonspecific proteases, predominates in the extracellular matrix of pliable tissues and organs, such as blood vessels, uterus, and gastrointestinal tract.

_____ 6. This component of the extracellular matrix accounts for the capacity of tissues to recoil after transient stretching.

_____ 7. This soluble plasma glycoprotein is also found in an insoluble form in tissues. Its specific binding sites allow it to bind to other extracellular matrix molecules, cells, and bacteria.

_____ 8. This glycoprotein is composed of six disulfide-linked subunits and is most abundant in perichondrium and tendons. During embryogenesis it has a modulatory function and is found in the dense extracellular matrix surrounding teeth buds, hair follicles, and mammary glands.

_____ 9. This extracellular matrix substance is composed of long, unbranched polysaccharide chains covalently bound to a protein core. Since they are hydrophilic, they maintain tissue turgor. Their high charge density accounts for the selective permeability of basement membranes.

_____ 10. These cell surface receptors are characterized by an RGD protein motif and mediate binding of cells to components of the extracellular matrix.

_____ 11. This small polypeptide is found in saliva and gastrointestinal secretions. It stimulates the proliferation of a variety of cells, thereby accelerating the healing of skin wounds and gastrointestinal ulcers. It also stimulates collagen deposition.

_____ 12. This cationic cytokine is released by macrophages, endothelial cells, platelets, and some other cells. It acts as a mitogen for mesenchymal cells, such as fibroblast, and smooth muscle cells.

_____ 13. This richly vascular connective tissue is found in the early stages of wound healing.

_____ 14. Sprouting of preexisting blood vessels under the influence of basic cytokines, such as fibroblast growth factor and vascular endothelial growth factor, results in the formation of new blood vessel.

_____ 15. It represents renewal of a lost tissue, in which the lost cells are replaced by identical ones.

_____ 16. This exuberant scar tends to enlarge on its own and recur after excision.

_____ 17. This granulation tissue cell is capable of contracting and synthesizing collagen.

_____ 18. This term denotes bursting of a wound because of inadequate healing.

_____ 19. This deformity of the palms results from abnormal healing of third-degree skin burns over the small hand joints.

_____ 20. Dupuytren contracture involving the palms, Ledderhose disease involving the plantae pedis, and Peyronie disease involving the penis are examples of this process.

DIRECTIONS: Choose the one best answer.

_____ 21. Vitamin C is required for which step in collagen synthesis?
   A. Hydroxylation of proline and lysine residues
   B. Glycosylation of the pro-α chains
   C. Chain association
   D. Disulfide bonding
   E. Triple-helix formation

_____ 22. Copper deficiency induced by nitrites, so-called lathyrism, is marked by collagen of low tensile strength, because collagen is not
   A. hydroxylated.
   B. glycosylated.
   C. cross-linked.
   D. disulfide-bonded.
   E. separated from the N-terminal propeptide.

_____ 23. In cycling cells, the main difference between rapidly dividing and slowly dividing cells is in the duration of which phase of the cell cycle?
   A. G_0
   B. G_1
   C. G_2
   D. S
   E. M

_____ 24. The replacement of dead cells cannot occur by regeneration in tissues composed of
   A. labile cells.
   B. stable cells.
   C. permanent cells.
   D. stem cells.
   E. embryonic cells.

_____ 25. Wound contraction is primarily mediated by
   A. smooth muscle cells.
   B. macrophages.
   C. fibroblasts.
   D. myofibroblasts.
   E. lymphocytes.

_____ 26. Sterile wound healing is characterized on day 4 by all the following *except*
   A. macrophages.
   B. polymorphonuclear leukocytes.
   C. capillary sprouts.
   D. fibroblasts.
   E. hyaluronic acid.

_____ 27. A healing wound reaches its maximal tensile strength
   A. at 2 weeks.
   B. at 6 weeks.
   C. at 3 months.
   D. at 1 year.
   E. over an unpredictable period of time.

_____ **28.** A mature scar differs from granulation tissue in that it has more
  A. cross-linked collagen.
  B. blood vessels.
  C. collagen type III.
  D. proteoglycans.
  E. fluid in the extracellular compartment.

_____ **29.** Regeneration typically occurs in all the following tissues *except*
  A. epidermis.
  B. liver.
  C. adrenal glands.
  D. kidney.
  E. lens.

_____ **30.** Factors that retard the healing of wounds include all the following *except*
  A. infection.
  B. ultraviolet light.
  C. lack of immobilization.
  D. diabetes mellitus.
  E. exogenous corticosteroids.

Answers

1. **The answer is C.** *Collagen type II* is found in cartilage but is also present in the vitreous humor of the eye and the nucleus pulposus of intervertebral discs.

2. **The answer is B.** *Collagen type I* is the major component of connective tissue in subcutaneous tissue and the skeleton.

3. **The answer is E.** *Collagen type IV*, a hydroxyproline-rich collagen of basement membranes, consists of triple helices interrupted by globular domains.

4. **The answer is M.** *Laminin*, a glycoprotein of basement membranes, has a cruciform (cross-like) structure. It mediates the adhesion of cells to basement membranes.

5. **The answer is D.** *Collagen type III* is a triple helix protein resistant to nonspecific proteases. It is typically found in the matrix of pliable tissues and organs, such as the blood vessels, uterus, and gastrointestinal tract.

6. **The answer is G.** *Elastic fibers* account for the capacity of tissues to recoil after stretching.

7. **The answer is I.** *Fibronectin* occurs in two forms: a soluble plasma form and an insoluble tissue form. It has numerous functions, but most notably it mediates adhesion between cells and tissue components.

8. **The answer is R.** *Tenascin* consists of six disulfide-linked units. It is formed in the perichondrium. During embryogenesis it plays a modulatory role in the formation of many organs.

9. **The answer is P.** *Proteoglycans* are composed of long, unbranched polysaccharide chains, constantly bound to a protein core. Proteoglycans

maintain tissue turgor and account for the selective permeability of basement membranes.

10. **The answer is K.** *Integrins* are cell surface receptors that contain an RGD (arginine-glycine-aspartate) protein sequence and mediate cell binding to collagens, laminin, and fibronectin.

11. **The answer is H.** *Epidermal growth factor* (EGF) was originally isolated from saliva, but it occurs in many other tissue fluids. It accelerates wound healing and stimulates collagen deposition, in addition to many other functions.

12. **The answer is O.** *Platelet-derived growth factor* (PDGF) was isolated from the α-granules of platelets. Later it was found in many other cells, including macrophages and endothelial cells. It binds to a receptor that is present on many mesenchymal cells and stimulates their division.

13. **The answer is J.** *Granulation tissue* is the term used to describe the aggregate of angioblasts (blood vessel cells), macrophages, and fibroblasts that fill the tissue defect in early stages of wound healing.

14. **The answer is A.** Formation of new blood vessels under the influence of cytokines is called *angiogenesis.*

15. **The answer is Q.** Renewal of lost cells or tissues by identical cells is termed *regeneration.*

16. **The answer is L.** Hypertrophic scars that do not regress are called *keloids.*

17. **The answer is N.** The *myofibroblast* has hybrid features of smooth muscle cells and fibroblasts and hence can both contract and lay down collagen.

18. **The answer is T.** Bursting of wounds due to inadequate healing is called *wound dehiscence.*

19. **The answer is F.** *Contractures* are caused by an abnormal connective-tissue response to injury or abnormal wound healing. They cause deformities of tissues, organs, or parts of the extremities.

20. **The answer is F.** Dupuytren contracture, Ledderhose disease, and Peyronie disease are clinical examples of *contractures.*

21. **The answer is A.** Vitamin C is required for the *hydroxylation of proline and lysine* prior to secretion of the collagen triple helix.

22. **The answer is C.** Copper is essential for the action of the metalloenzyme lysyl oxidase, an enzyme that mediates the cross-linking of collagen by promoting the formation of intramolecular and intermolecular bonds. This process establishes the tensile strength of collagen fibers.

23. **The answer is B.** The main difference between rapidly and slowly dividing cells is in the duration of the G_1 (Gap 1) *phase.* In cycling cells, this phase occurs immediately after mitosis has been completed. During G_1, the cell is devoted to specialized activities, which vary from one cell type to another.

24. **The answer is C.** The loss of *permanent cells,* such as neurons, cannot be replaced by regeneration because the remaining neurons cannot enter mitosis. On the other hand, the loss of hepatocytes, which are stable

cells, is compensated for by the reentry of other hepatocytes into the mitotic cycle.

25. **The answer is D.** *Myofibroblasts*, cells with features intermediate between fibroblasts and smooth muscle cells, appear in the wound 2 to 3 days after injury. Their active contraction decreases the size of the defect.

26. **The answer is B.** Uninfected wounds do not display polymorphonuclear leukocytes (PMNs), except during the earliest stages (first 2 days) of the removal of tissue debris. The presence of PMNs in the wound and frank pus formation after day 3 are signs of infection. Granulation tissue contains fibroblasts, angioblasts, macrophages, and extracellular matrix. Hyaluronic acid, owing to its hydrophilic properties, accounts for swelling and water retention in the wound.

27. **The answer is E.** The tensile strength of a wound is variable and depends on the circumstances. Age, the presence of infection, nutritional status, and the size of the tissue defect all influence the rate at which tensile strength develops. Tensile strength increases slowly, even after the amount of collagen accumulated has reached its maximum.

28. **The answer is A.** A mature scar is typically composed of *cross-linked collagen*, which has replaced the early components of extracellular matrix in a healing wound. During the formation of a scar, blood vessels in the richly vascular granulation tissue are progressively obliterated. The elimination of hydrophilic proteoglycans reduces the water-binding capacity of the tissue.

29. **The answer is E.** The lens is composed of postmitotic permanent cells, which cannot regenerate.

30. **The answer is B.** Ultraviolet light accelerates wound healing, whereas all the other factors listed retard it.

Chapter 4

Immunopathology

Questions

DIRECTIONS: Match each numbered statement with the most appropriate lettered item. Each lettered item can be used once, more than once, or not at all.

Immune-Mediated Diseases

A. AIDS
B. Allergic rhinitis
C. Amyloidosis
D. Asthma
E. Dermatomyositis
F. DiGeorge syndrome
G. Erythroblastosis fetalis
H. Goodpasture syndrome
I. Graft-versus-host disease
J. Graves' disease
K. Isolated IgA deficiency
L. Mixed connective-tissue disease
M. Myasthenia gravis
N. Polymyositis
O. Severe combined immunodeficiency
P. Sjögren syndrome
Q. Systemic lupus erythematosus
R. Systemic sclerosis (scleroderma)
S. Wiskott-Aldrich syndrome
T. X-linked agammaglobulinemia of Bruton

_____ 1. An 8-month-old boy with recurrent bacterial pneumonia was found to have almost no IgG in the blood. Cell-mediated immunity was normal. His brother had the same disease and died of echovirus encephalitis. His parents and two sisters were normal.

_____ 2. A 40-year-old woman complained of a dry mouth and dry eyes and had difficulty swallowing bread and meat. The physician noticed a preauricular tender mass on the left side. Serologic tests revealed antinuclear antibodies (ANA) and antibodies to ribonucleoproteins SS-A and SS-B.

_____ 3. A 35-year-old woman complained of intermittent blanching of the fingers, associated with tingling and pain upon exposure to cold. She also noted tightness of skin around her mouth and had problems swallowing food. On physical examination the doctor noticed a "stone face" and sclerodactyly.

_____ 4. Antibodies to topoisomerase I and centromeres were detected in a woman with renal failure and hypertension of recent origin.

_____ 5. Ocular muscle weakness and general fatigability were found in a 35-year-old woman, who also had antibodies to acetylcholine receptors.

_____ 6. An edematous jaundiced baby was born to an Rh⁻ woman who had anti-Rh antibodies.

_____ 7. This disease is characterized by episodes of coughing, wheezing, and shortness of breath. Leukotrienes play a major pathogenetic role by causing contraction of smooth muscle cells.

_____ 8. Fibrinoid necrosis of glomerular capillaries and mesangial cell proliferation were seen in a kidney biopsy of a 40-year-old woman with microscopic hematuria and proteinuria. Antinuclear antibodies (ANA) were present in a titer of 1:256. Antibodies to double-stranded DNA and Sm antigen were present in a titer of 1:128.

_____ 9. A 25-year-old woman complained of low-grade fever, fatigue, and persistent rash over her nose and upper chest. She also had pains in her knees and elbows and anemia. A skin biopsy revealed dermal inflammation and granular deposits of IgG and C3 complement along the basement membrane at the epidermal/dermal junction. Urinalysis revealed microscopic hematuria and proteinuria. The ANA test was positive.

_____ 10. Sweating, tachycardia, weight loss, and exophthalmos were noted in a 50-year-old woman. Her thyroid was enlarged and warm on palpation. The blood level of thyroid stimulating hormone (TSH) was low, and the levels of thyroid hormones T_3 and T_4 were elevated.

_____ 11. This most common type I hypersensitivity disease in adults presents with nasal congestion and bouts of sneezing.

_____ 12. This most common inborn immunodeficiency is often asymptomatic.

_____ 13. This x-linked, recessive, congenital immunodeficiency characterized by recurrent infections, edema, and bleeding due to thrombocytopenia was diagnosed in a 2-year-old child.

_____ 14. Skin rash, diarrhea, and jaundice were noticed in a leukemic patient treated with total body irradiation and bone marrow transplantation.

_____ 15. Adenosine deaminase deficiency was diagnosed in a 9-month-old child. It was associated with a virtual absence of lymphocytes from the thymus, spleen, and lymph nodes.

_____ 16. Congenital aplasia of the thymus and parathyroid glands was diagnosed in a neonate that developed spastic contraction on the second postpartum day.

_____ **17.** A 50-year-old woman was found to have fever, myositis, Raynaud phenomenon, anemia, lymphadenopathy, and hypergammaglob-ulinemia. The ANA test was positive in high titer, but there was no evidence of anti-double DNA and anti-Sm antibodies. Urinalysis was normal. The patient responded well to steroids.

_____ **18.** *Pneumocystis carinii* pneumonia was diagnosed in a 40-year-old man with lymphopenia and a CD-4 cell count of 120/µL.

_____ **19.** Kaposi sarcoma and lymphoma of the brain were diagnosed in a 30-year-old homosexual man.

_____ **20.** This systemic disease was diagnosed at autopsy. The liver, kid-neys, spleen and adrenals were infiltrated with eosinophilic extracellular, insoluble material that reacted with Congo red.

DIRECTIONS: Choose the one best answer.

_____ **21.** Which of the following is true for CD4+ lymphocytes?
A. They account for less than one-third of peripheral T-lympho-cytes in the blood and lymphoid organs.
B. They have suppressor functions.
C. They secrete interleukin-2.
D. They are cytotoxic.
E. They secrete lgE.

_____ **22.** Which of the following is true for natural killer cells?
A. They may phagocytose tumor cells.
B. Killing of cells is enhanced by interleukin-2.
C. They recognize and kill some virus-infected cells.
D. Killing of cells is stimulated by prostaglandin E_2.
E. Killing of cells requires interaction with B cells.

_____ **23.** Macrophages secrete all the following *except*
A. interleukin-1.
B. tumor necrosis factor.
C. arachidonic acid derivatives.
D. plasminogen activator.
E. kappa chains of immunoglobulins.

_____ **24.** Class I molecules of the major histocompatibility complex
A. consist of an α and β chain glycoprotein.
B. express two antigens codominantly for each locus.
C. are expressed primarily on macrophages and B cells.
D. are recognized by NK cells.
E. are lipoproteins.

_____ **25.** Hypersensitivity reaction involving IgE antibody production and mast cells is called
A. type I, anaphylactic reaction.
B. type II, cytotoxic reaction.
C. type III, immune complex-mediated reaction.
D. type IV, delayed-type hypersensitivity reaction.
E. graft versus host reaction.

_____ **26.** All the following conditions represent a type II hypersensitivity
reaction *except*
  A. autoimmune hemolytic anemia.
  B. myasthenia gravis.
  C. transfusion reaction.
  D. Graves disease.
  E. hay fever.

_____ **27.** Immune complex-mediated (type III hypersensitivity) reaction
causes tissue lesions in
  A. polyarteritis nodosa.
  B. pemphigus vulgaris.
  C. bullous pemphigoid.
  D. poison ivy reaction.
  E. chronic renal graft rejection.

_____ **28.** Hyperacute renal transplant rejection is mediated by
  A. T-helper lymphocytes.
  B. T-suppressor lymphocytes.
  C. NK cells.
  D. IgE.
  E. complement.

Answers

1. **The answer is T.** *X-linked agammaglobulinemia of Bruton* is a sex-linked
recessive disorder that affects boys and typically presents by the end of
the first year of life with recurrent bacterial infections. The disease is
caused by a mutation of the gene encoding a tyrosine kinase that is
essential for B-cell maturation into plasma cells. Since plasma cells are
not formed, no immunoglobulins are produced, and the patients typically succumb to bacterial infections. T-cell defense is intact, protecting
the affected boys from most viruses except for a few pathogens such as
echovirus, which may cause fatal encephalitis.

2. **The answer is P.** *Sjögren disease* is an autoimmune disorder that typically
presents with chronic inflammation of the lacrimal and salivary glands.
Sjögren disease may occur in the course of generalized autoimmune diseases such as systemic lupus erythematosus (SLE) (secondary Sjögren
disease) or in an isolated form (primary Sjögren disease). Dacryocystitis
and sialadenitis present clinically as xerophthalmia (dry eyes) or xerostomia (dry mouth), respectively. Sjögren disease may cause enlargement
of salivary glands, so-called Mikulicz syndrome. In such cases a biopsy
must be performed to exclude other causes of Mikulicz syndrome, such
as sarcoidosis or lymphoma. Serologic tests (e.g. rheumatoid factor and
ANA) are positive in most cases. However, they are not useful for dis-
tinguishing primary Sjögren disease from the secondary Sjögren disease
encountered in rheumatoid arthritis, SLE, or systemic sclerosis. Antiri-
bonucleoprotein antibodies (SS-A and SS-B) are almost diagnostic of primary Sjögren disease but are not encountered in secondary Sjögren disease.

3. **The answer is R.** CREST syndrome is an acronym describing the features of a mild form of *systemic sclerosis,* which is limited to the skin of the face and fingers and shows late involvement of internal organs, predominantly the esophagus. The acronym stands for *c*alcinosis, *R*aynaud phenomenon, *e*sophageal dysmotility, *s*clerodactyly, and *t*elangiectasia.

4. **The answer is R.** *Systemic sclerosis* typically presents with antibodies to DNA topoisomerase I or the centromeres of chromosomes. Antibodies to DNA topoisomerase I (anti-Scl 70) are typical of diffuse scleroderma, whereas anti-centromere antibodies are diagnostic of CREST syndrome.

5. **The answer is M.** *Myasthenia gravis* is a type II hypersensitivity disorder caused by antibodies that bind to acetylcholine receptors. These antibodies interfere with the transmission of neural impulses at the neuromuscular junction, causing muscle weakness and easy fatigability. External ocular and eyelid muscles are most often affected, but the disease is often progressive and may cause death by respiratory muscle paralysis.

6. **The answer is G.** *Erythroblastosis fetalis* is a hemolytic disease caused in the Rh^+ fetus by maternal anti-Rh IgG. Typically, the antibodies to Rh antigen develop in an Rh^- mother sensitized by the blood of her Rh^+ fetus during delivery. If the subsequent pregnancy results in another Rh^+ fetus, the maternal anti-Rh IgG can cross the placenta and cause a hemolytic disease in the intrauterine fetus. Erythroblastosis fetalis presents with jaundice and edema caused by massive hemolysis.

7. **The answer is D.** *Asthma* associated with extrinsic allergens is triggered by IgE attached to mast cells in the bronchial mucosa. The release of histamine and other mast cell–derived mediators causes bronchospasm and mucous secretion and initiates a persistent inflammation in the bronchial wall. Leukotrienes, also known as slow-reacting substances of anaphylaxis (SRS-A), are generated from arachidonic acid in this inflammatory process and are thought to be the most important chemical mediators of asthma.

8. **The answer is Q.** *Systemic lupus erythmatosus* (SLE) often presents with proliferative glomerulonephritis. In such cases, the glomeruli may also display fibrinoid necrosis of blood vessels. The diagnosis of SLE is based on the typical serologic findings. Antibodies to double-stranded DNA (positive in 50% of SLE patients) and to Sm antigen (positive in 25% of SLE patients) are diagnostic. Antinuclear antibodies (ANA) are less specific and occur not only in SLE but also in other autoimmune diseases. The ANA test is an inexpensive and sensitive test that is useful for screening and the initial diagnosis of autoimmune diseases.

9. **The answer is Q.** *Systemic lupus erythmatosus* (SLE) is a multisystemic autoimmune disease that often presents with fever, fatigue, skin rash, joint pain, and renal symptoms. Fatigue is in part due to anemia and in part due to the action of cytokines (e.g., TNF, IL-1). The latter are released in the course of the inflammation caused by antigen/antibody complex deposition in various tissues.

10. **The answer is J.** *Graves disease* is a type II hypersensitivity disorder caused by antibodies to the TSH receptor on follicular cells of the thyroid. Antibody binding to the TSH receptor stimulates a release of tetraiodothyronine (T_4) and triiodothyronine (T_3) from the thyroid into the circulation. Circulating T_4 and T_3 suppress TSH production in the pituitary. Sweating, weight loss, and tachycardia are evidence of the

hypermetabolism typical of hyperthyroidism. Graves' disease also causes exophthalmos (bulging eyes).

11. **The answer is B.** *Allergic rhinitis* (hay fever) is the most common type I hypersensitivity disease in adults. It may be caused by pollen, house dust, animal dandruff, and many other allergens. Antigens inhaled in the air react with the IgE attached to the basophils in the nasal mucosa, thereby triggering the release of vasoactive substances stored in the mast cell granules. Histamine, the main mediator released from mast cells, increases the permeability of mucosal vessels, causing edema and sneezing.

12. **The answer is K.** *Isolated IgA deficiency* is a genetic disorder that occurs at a rate of 1:60 in the general population. Although it is often asymptomatic, it may present with recurrent upper respiratory or intestinal infections. A significant number of these patients have antibodies to IgA and may react unfavorably if transfused with normal blood that contains IgA.

13. **The answer is S.** *Wiskott-Aldrich syndrome* is a complex X-linked disease characterized clinically by a triad of recurrent infections, eczema, and thrombocytopenia. The peripheral T-cell zones of the lymph nodes are depleted of lymphocytes, even though the thymus is usually normal. These patients are at an increased risk for lymphoma.

14. **The answer is I.** *Graft-versus-host reaction* presents with skin rash, diarrhea, and jaundice. These symptoms are caused by the donor's T-lymphocytes, which are transferred to an immunosuppressed patient together with other hemtopoietic cells during bone marrow transplantation. The donor's T-lymphocytes recognize the host tissues as foreign and react by destroying the host's cells. The gastrointestinal mucosa, epidermis, and intrahepatic bile ducts are most often affected.

15. **The answer is O.** *Severe combined immunodeficiency* of T and B cells is a heterogeneous group of disorders. About one-half of these severely immunodeficient children lack adenosine deaminase (ADA). ADA deficiency causes the accumulation of toxic intermediate products, such as deoxyadenosine, which are toxic to lymphocytes. Neither T nor B-lymphocytes are formed under such conditions. These children cannot survive beyond early infancy, unless raised in an entirely sterile environment ("bubble children").

16. **The answer is F.** *DiGeorge syndrome* is a chromosomal genetic defect that results in developmental anomalies of the branchial (pharyngeal) pouches and the organs that develop from these embryonic structures (thymus, parathyroids, and the aortic arch). These children present with tetany caused by hypoparathyroidism and T-lymphocyte deficiency. They also have characteristic facial features ("angry look") and vascular abnormalities of the aortic arch.

17. **The answer is L.** *Mixed connective-tissue disease* (MCTD) has some features of SLE, polymyositis, or scleroderma but is distinct from these diseases. Renal disease rarely occurs. Patients typically have high levels of antibodies that react with ribonucleoproteins; the ANA test is positive. However, unlike SLE patients, they do not have antibodies to Sm antigen or native (double-stranded) DNA. MCTD responds well to corticosteroids.

18. **The answer is A.** *Pneumocystis carinii* is one of the diseases that defines AIDS. Unless the immunodeficiency is related to cytotoxic therapy, one should assume that such a pneumonia is a sign of *AIDS*.

19. **The answer is A.** Kaposi sarcoma and brain lymphoma in middle-aged adults are typical complications of *AIDS*.

20. **The answer is C.** *Amyloidosis* is a systemic disease characterized by the deposition of a fibrillar protein known as amyloid. It stains with Congo red and has typical electron microscopic features.

21. **The answer is C.** CD4$^+$ lymphocytes, also known as T-helper cells, constitute 65% of all peripheral lymphocytes. They regulate immune functions by secreting helper molecules such as *interleukin-2*. Suppressor and cytotoxic functions are performed by CD8$^+$ lymphocytes (T-suppressor lymphocytes). Immunoglobulins are secreted by B-lymphocytes and plasma cells.

22. **The answer is B.** Natural killer (NK) cells recognize and kill some tumor cells and virus-infected cells but do not phagocytose them. *Interleukin-2* promotes and prostaglandin E$_2$ suppresses the activity of NK cells. NK cells do not require B-cell cooperation, and they act without previous sensitization.

23. **The answer is E.** Macrophages secrete interleukin-1, tumor necrosis factor, alpha interferon, angiogenesis factor, arachidonic acid derivatives (prostaglandin E2, prostacycline, thromboxanes, leukotrienes), and various enzymes (e.g., plasminogen activator). They do not synthesize *immoglobulins*.

24. **The answer is B.** Class I MHC molecules are glycoproteins, not lipoproteins. They consist of a single, transmembranous, heavy chain associated with a constant surface molecule, called α_2-microglobulin. By contrast, class II MHC molecules consist of two transmembranous glycoproteins, the α and β chains. Alleles for each locus are expressed codominantly (i.e., *antigen* inherited from each parent is expressed equally). All tissues express class I molecules, whereas class II molecules are displayed primarily on macrophages and B cells. Class I antigens are recognized by cytotoxic T cells and play a major role in graft rejection and the killing of virus-infected cells.

25. **The answer is A.** The *type I anaphylactic reaction* is mediated by IgE, whereas types II and III are mediated by IgG or IgM. Delayed-type hypersensitivity and graft-versus-host reaction do not involve antibody production but are mediated by T-lymphocytes, with the help of macrophages.

26. **The answer is E.** Type II hypersensitivity reaction is mediated by antibodies binding to the cell surface of target cells. In hemolytic anemia and transfusion reactions, the destruction of red blood cells is mediated by cytotoxic IgG or IgM antibodies. Antibodies to acetylcholine receptors at the neuromuscular junction cause myasthenia gravis. Goodpasture syndrome is caused by antibodies to the globular domain of collagen type IV. Antibodies to the thyroid-stimulating hormone (TSH) receptor cause Graves' disease. *Hay fever* is an IgE-mediated type I hypersensitivity reaction.

27. **The answer is A.** Local formation of immune complexes in the walls of blood vessels is the primary pathogenetic mechanism for *polyarteritis*

nodosa. By contrast, in pemphigus antibodies directly attack epidermal cells of the skin. In bullous pemphigoid antibodies attack the basement membrane at the epidermal/dermal interface rather than form circulating immune complexes. Pemphigus and pemphigoid are thus based on a type II hypersensitivity (cytotoxic) reaction. Poison ivy skin reaction and chronic renal graft rejections are cell-mediated (type IV) hypersensitivity reactions.

28. **The answer is E.** Hyperacute renal graft rejection is mediated by preexisting circulating antibodies to the graft in the recipient. These antibodies activate *complement* and the coagulation system.

Chapter 5

Neoplasia

Questions

DIRECTIONS: Match each numbered description of a specific tumor with the most appropriate lettered item from the list of suggested diagnoses. Each lettered item may be used once, more than once, or not at all.

Neoplasms

    A. Adenocarcinoma
    B. Adenoma
    C. Burkitt lymphoma
    D. Chronic myelogenous leukemia
    E. Ewing sarcoma
    F. Glioblastoma multiforme
    G. Kaposi sarcoma
    H. Leiomyoma
    I. Leiomyosarcoma
    J. Lipoma
    K. Malignant melanoma
    L. Meningioma
    M. Mesothelioma
    N. Retinoblastoma
    O. Rhabdomyosarcoma
    P. Schwannoma
    Q. Squamous cell carcinoma
    R. Teratoma
    S. Transitional cell carcinoma
    T. Wilms' tumor

1. Multiple, pedunculated, benign tumors in the colon of a 10-year-old boy

2. Bilateral eye tumor in a 2-year-old child

3. Benign, soft, yellow tumor of subcutaneous tissue

4. Benign, primary, intracranial tumor attached to the dura

5. Hemorrhagic cutaneous nodules in a male homosexual with AIDS

E   **6.** Primary malignant bone tumor in the diaphysis of the tibia in a 12-year-old boy

H   **7.** Benign tumor of the myometrium in a 40-year-old woman

L   **8.** Benign ovarian tumor composed of tissues derived from all three primary germ layers removed from a 20-year-old woman

F   **9.** Primary malignant brain tumor in a 60-year-old man

M   **10.** Pleural tumor in a retired pipefitter who worked in a shipyard during World War II

K   **11.** Pigmented eye tumor in a 50-year-old man

   12. Malignant tumor originating from the muscular layers of the stomach

O   **13.** Malignant tumor of the thigh composed of striated muscle cells

S   **14.** The most common malignant epithelial urinary bladder tumor

C   **15.** Malignant tumor of the jaw related to Epstein-Barr virus in an 8-year-old African girl

t   **16.** Malignant renal tumor in a 4-year-old boy

P   **17.** Benign subcutaneous tumor attached to peripheral nerve

Q   **18.** Carcinoma of the larynx in a 60-year-old smoker

A   **19.** Malignant tumor of the pancreas causing jaundice

D   **20.** Hemopoietic malignancy that exhibits the Philadelphia chromosome

---

DIRECTIONS: Match the following numbered tumors with the most appropriate lettered item. Each lettered item can be used once, more than once, or not at all.

Tumor Markers

   A. α-Fetoprotein (AFP)
   B. Carcinoembryonic antigen (CEA)
   C. Chromogranin
   D. Chorionic gonadotropin (hCG)
   E. Coagulation factor VIII
   F. Desmin
   G. Glial fibrillary acidic protein
   H. Immunoglobulin
   I. Leukocyte common antigen

B   **21.** Adenocarcinoma of the colon

C   **22.** Islet cell carcinoma of the pancreas

F   **23.** Leiomyoma

A   **24.** Hepatocellular carcinoma

A   **25.** Yolk sac carcinoma of the ovary

Environmental Carcinogens

A. Aflatoxin B
B. Aniline dyes
C. Asbestos
D. Nitrosamines
E. Polycyclic aromatic hydrocarbons
F. Ultraviolet light
G. Vinyl chloride

C   **26.** Mesothelioma

E   **27.** Scrotal cancer

E   **28.** Lung cancer in smokers

B   **29.** Bladder cancer

G   **30.** Angiosarcoma of liver

Highest Incidence of Specific Cancers

A. China
B. India
C. Japan
D. Uganda
E. United States

E   **31.** Colorectal cancer

C   **32.** Stomach cancer

A   **33.** Nasopharyngeal carcinoma

E   **34.** Breast cancer

E   **35.** Prostatic cancer

D   **36.** Burkitt lymphoma

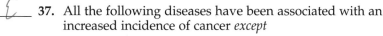

DIRECTIONS: Choose the one best answer.

E   **37.** All the following diseases have been associated with an increased incidence of cancer *except*

A. cirrhosis caused by hepatitis B virus.
B. ulcerative colitis.
C. dysplasia of bronchial epithelium.
D. leukoplakia of oral mucosa.
E. osteoporosis.

A   **38.** Chromosomal changes known as homogeneous staining regions and extrachromosomal double minutes are typically associated with oncogene

A. amplification.
B. inactivation.
C. transduction.
D. mutation.
E. deletion.

39. A pathologist was asked to evaluate the N-*myc* oncogene in a tumor of a 5-year-old child because this test might provide important prognostic data. The tumor involved both adrenals and several long bones and was composed of "small blue cells" with a high nucleus-to-cytoplasm ratio. This tumor is most likely a

A. teratoma.
B. retinoblastoma.
C. neuroblastoma.
D. medulloblastoma.
E. small cell carcinoma of the lung.

40. An 8-year-old girl with numerous hypopigmented, ulcerated, and crusted patches on her face and forearms developed an indurated, crater-like, skin nodule on the back of her left hand. Biopsy disclosed a squamous cell carcinoma of the skin. A molecular biology study disclosed a mutation of a gene encoding a nucleotide excision repair enzyme. This girl has

A. xeroderma pigmentosum.
B. ataxia telangiectasia.
C. hereditary albinism.
D. neurofibromatosis, type I.
E. Li-Fraumeni syndrome.

41. Staging of tumors is based on

A. clinical assessment of tumor size and spread.
B. histologic assessment of tumor differentiation.
C. cytologic assessment of nuclear features.
D. multimodal assessment of anaplasia.
E. tumor classification.

42. Seeding of tumor cells within abdominal cavity is particularly characteristic of cancer of which organ?

A. Testis
B. Ovary
C. Uterus
D. Vagina
E. Prostate

43. The most common malignant neoplasm among men in the United States is cancer of which organ?

A. Lung
B. Stomach
C. Colon
D. Prostate
E. Testis

44. The most common cause of cancer-related death among men and women in the United States is cancer of which organ?

A. Lung
B. Breast
C. Pancreas
D. Colon
E. Urinary bladder

E

_____ **45.** Which of the following neoplasms has been linked to a deletion of a tumor suppressor gene?
- A. Hepatocellular carcinoma
- B. Chondrosarcoma
- C. Glioblastoma multiforme
- D. Medulloblastoma
- E. Retinoblastoma

A n s w e r s

1. **The answer is B.** The large intestine of young people with familial adenomatous polyposis coli is studded with numerous tubular or villous *adenomas*. These benign tumors have a tendency to undergo malignant transformation, which usually occurs later in adulthood.

2. **The answer is N.** *Retinoblastomas* are malignant ocular tumors of young children. They are bilateral in 15% of cases.

3. **The answer is J.** *Lipomas* are benign tumors of subcutaneous soft tissue. Because they are composed of fat cells, these tumors appear yellow on cross section. Lipomas may also occur in other sites containing fat cells (e.g., retroperitoneum, omentum). Malignant adipose cell tumors are called liposarcomas.

4. **The answer is L.** *Meningiomas* are benign intracranial tumors that originate from the dura mater. They are typically attached to the dura and compress the brain.

5. **The answer is G.** *Kaposi sarcoma* is a malignant tumor of endothelial cells, which may occur in a sporadic or epidemic form. Epidemic Kaposi sarcoma, linked to infection with herpesvirus, type 8, affects male homosexuals suffering from AIDS. The tumors present as hemorrhagic skin nodules.

6. **The answer is E.** *Ewing sarcoma* is a malignant bone tumor of young people, which tends to occur in the diaphysis of long bones. The cell of origin and the histogenesis of this tumor are controversial.

7. **The answer is H.** *Leiomyoma* is the most common benign tumor of the uterus, usually arising in women of reproductive age. It originates from the smooth muscle cells of the myometrium.

8. **The answer is R.** *Teratomas* are benign tumors composed of tissues derived from all three primary germ layers, ectoderm, mesoderm, and endoderm. They are most common in the ovary but also occur in the testis and extragonadal sites.

9. **The answer is F.** *Glioblastoma multiforme* is the most common malignant primary brain tumor. It is composed of neoplastic glial cells corresponding to anaplastic astrocytes.

10. **The answer is M.** *Mesothelioma* is a malignant tumor of the pleura and peritoneum, which has been causally linked to occupational exposure to asbestos. This fibrous silicate has been used for insulating pipes. The pipefitters working in shipyards were the most exposed workers. Many of these workers developed mesotheliomas 20–30 years after exposure.

11. **The answer is K.** *Malignant melanoma* is a pigmented eye tumor originating from melanocytes of the iris or retina. Melanomas of the skin are more common than the eye tumors.

12. **The answer is I.** *Leiomyosarcomas* are malignant tumors that originate from the smooth muscle layers of the stomach or intestines. Histologically, they are indistinguishable from other smooth muscle cell tumors such as leiomyosarcomas.

13. **The answer is O.** *Rhabdomyosarcoma* is a malignant tumor of striated muscle. It occurs in muscles of the thigh or at any other muscular sites. The tumor has a peak incidence in childhood.

14. **The answer is S.** *Transitional cell carcinoma* is the most common malignant tumor of the urinary bladder, an organ normally lined by transitional epithelium. Only 10% of urinary bladder tumors are squamous cell carcinomas, which are preceded by squamous metaplasia.

15. **The answer is C.** Endemic *Burkitt lymphoma* is most prevalent in sub-Saharan Africa and is related to infection with Epstein-Barr virus. These lymphomas tend to be extranodal (i.e., they do not originate in lymph nodes). The hemopoietic bone marrow of the jaws is often involved. These tumors grow rapidly and cause massive facial disfiguration.

16. **The answer is T.** *Wilms tumor* (nephroblastoma) is the most common renal tumor of infants and children. Histologically, it is composed of immature tubules and mesenchymal cells ("blastoma") resembling the renal primordium or fetal kidney. It is linked to a loss or mutation of tumor suppressor gene (WT-1). Wilms' tumor may be sporadic or familial, one-sided or bilateral (10%).

17. **The answer is P.** *Schwannoma* (neurilemmoma) is a benign tumor originating from Schwann cells that envelop peripheral nerves.

18. **The answer is Q.** Cancers of the larynx, especially those arising in cigarette smokers, are almost all classified histologically as *squamous cell carcinomas*.

19. **The answer is A.** Most cancers of the pancreas are histologically classified as *adenocarcinomas*, which originate from the pancreatic ducts. Tumors of the head of the pancreas tend to obstruct the common bile duct and cause extrahepatic jaundice.

20. **The answer is D.** *Chronic myelogenous leukemia* originates from hemopoietic cells in the bone marrow. The leukemic cells show a chromosomal translocation that results in shortening of the chromosome. This chromosome, a marker of CML, is known as the Philadelphia chromosome.

21. **The answer is B.** *Adenocarcinomas* of the colon usually express carcinoembryonic antigen (CEA), a glycoprotein that is released into the circulation and serves as a serologic marker for these tumors. CEA is also found in association with other gastrointestinal cancers and malignant tumors of the pancreas, and even those of the lung or ovary. Elevated serum levels of CEA also occur in patients with chronic ulcerative colitis and even in some disease-free persons, especially if they are smokers. Thus, the usefulness of this tumor marker for the screening and detection of early neoplasia of the colon is limited.

22. **The answer is C.** Islet cell carcinomas of the pancreas contain cytoplasmic neuroendocrine granules rich in the matrix protein *chromogranin*.

However, since such granules occur in all neuroendocrine cells, this marker is not specific for insulinomas and does not distinguish pancreatic from extrapancreatic neuroendocrine neoplasms.

23. **The answer is F.** Leiomyomas are smooth muscle cell tumors that, like all muscle cells in the body, contain intermediate filaments rich in *desmin*.

24. **The answer is A.** *α-Fetoprotein* (AFP) is normally produced during fetal life by cells that form the yolk sac (an extraembryonic structure that atrophies during intrauterine development) and by liver cells. By contrast, adult liver cells do not produce AFP. Elevation of serum AFP is in most cases associated with tumors that contain yolk sac cells or transformed hepatocytes.

25. **The answer is A.** Yolk sac carcinomas are germ cell–derived tumors most commonly located in the testis or the ovary. As previously noted, they may produce *AFP*.

26. **The answer is C.** Mesothelioma has been linked to industrial exposure to *asbestos*.

27. **The answer is E.** Scrotal cancer in chimney sweeps, the first cancer causally related to an environmental carcinogen, was a consequence of exposure to coal tar, which contained *polycyclic aromatic hydrocarbons*.

28. **The answer is E.** Lung cancer is mostly due to smoking, probably because tobacco also contains *polycyclic aromatic hydrocarbons*. Asbestos-related lung disease seems to potentiate the carcinogenic effects of smoking.

29. **The answer is B.** The incidence of bladder cancer is increased in *aniline dye workers*. The azo dyes are converted to watersoluble carcinogens in the liver and are excreted in the urine, where they primarily affect the surface epithelium of the bladder.

30. **The answer is G.** *Vinyl chloride* is used in the rubber industry and has been linked to the development of angiosarcoma of the liver.

31. **The answer is E.** The reasons for the geographic variation in the incidence of various forms of cancer are poorly understood and are mostly hypothetical. The high incidence of colorectal cancer in the *United States* is theoretically linked to diet, specifically high in fat and low in fiber intake.

32. **The answer is C.** Diet has been blamed for the high incidence of gastric cancer in *Japan*, although it also may be related to the common occurrence of atrophic gastritis in that country.

33. **The answer is A.** It has been proposed that the high prevalence of nasopharyngeal carcinoma in *China* reflects Epstein-Barr virus infection, but this hypothesis remains unproved.

34. **The answer is E.** It is not known why American women are at a higher risk of developing breast cancer than Asian women. Since women of Japanese extraction living in the *United States* appear to be at a higher risk for this tumor than those in Japan, environmental factors are thought to play a role.

35. **The answer is E.** Prostatic cancer is a tumor of old age, and its increased incidence is most likely related to the prolonged lifespan in the *United States* and in other countries of the Western world.

36. **The answer is D.** Burkitt lymphoma is common in Central Africa, whereas it is uncommon and sporadic in other continents. This lymphoid malignancy accounts for half of all tumors in *Uganda*.

37. **The answer is E.** Cirrhosis and chronic hepatitis caused by hepatitis B virus are associated with an increased incidence of hepatocellular carcinoma. Ulcerative colitis predisposes to adenocarcinoma of the large intestine. Bronchial dysplasia, typically found in smokers, leads to squamous cell carcinoma of the bronchi. Leukoplakia of the mouth may progress to oral carcinoma. *Osteoporosis* is, however, not a premalignant condition.

38. **The answer is A.** Homogeneous staining regions (HSR) and extrachromosal double minutes are signs of oncogene *amplification*.

39. **The answer is C.** Amplification of the N-*myc* oncogene is found in treatment-resistant *neuroblastomas* that have a poor prognosis.

40. **The answer is A.** *Xeroderma pigmentosum* is an autosomal recessive disorder related to mutations of genes that encode DNA-repair enzymes. Affected persons are extremely sensitive to skin injury produced by UV radiation and develop skin cancer at an early age.

41. **The answer is A.** Staging of tumors is based on the *clinical and x-ray assessment of tumor size and spread*. Grading of tumors is based on histologic assessment of its differentiation.

42. **The answer is B.** Peritoneal seeding is a feature of *ovarian carcinomas*.

43. **The answer is D.** Carcinoma of the *prostate* is the most common tumor in men.

44. **The answer is A.** *Lung carcinoma* is the cause of most cancer-related deaths in the United States and most countries of Western Europe.

45. **The answer is E.** *Retinoblastoma* is pathogenetically related to the deletion of a segment of chromosome 13, which normally contains the Rb gene. The deletion of the chromosome fragment 13q14 can be recognized in karyograms of retinoblastoma cells.

Chapter 6

Developmental and Genetic Disorders

DIRECTIONS: Match each numbered statement with the most appropriate lettered item. Each lettered item can be used once, more than once, or not at all.

A. Achondroplasia
B. Anencephaly
C. Cephalohematoma
D. Cleft palate
E. Cystic fibrosis
F. Down syndrome
G. Duchenne muscular dystrophy
H. Ehlers-Danlos syndrome
I. Erythroblastosis fetalis
J. Familial hypercholesterolemia
K. Fragile-X syndrome
L. Hemophilia
M. Klinefelter syndrome
N. Marfan syndrome
O. Neurofibromatosis, type I
P. Osteogenesis imperfecta
Q. Phenylketonuria
R. Spina bifida
S. Tay-Sachs disease
T. Turner syndrome

_____ 1. Infertile male with a 47,XXY karyotype

_____ 2. Short woman with primary amenorrhea and a 45,X karyotype

_____ 3. Mental retardation and enlarged testicles, associated with amplification of *CCG* triple nucleotide repeats on the X chromosome

_____ 4. Recurrent hemarthrosis in a 12-year-old boy, whose brother has the same disease

_____ 5. Dwarfism characterized by short legs and arms and a normal-sized head, inherited as an autosomal dominant trait

_____ 6. Multiple fractures and blue sclerae in a neonate

_____ **7.** Meconium ileus

_____ **8.** Autosomal dominant disease caused by a mutation of the gene encoding the low density lipoprotein (LDL) receptor

_____ **9.** Autosomal recessive disease causing mental deficiency if the infant is not given a special diet

_____ **10.** Polygenic dysraphic disorder characterized by a defect in or incomplete formation of vertebral arches

_____ **11.** Lethal lysosomal storage disease that presents at an early age with progressive mental deterioration and blindness

_____ **12.** Central nervous system malformation associated with incomplete development of the calvaria and incompatible with life

_____ **13.** Lethal X-linked hereditary disease that typically causes elevation of creatine kinase in the amniotic fluid

_____ **14.** Polygenic disorder affecting the development of the mouth, which is more common in males than in females

_____ **15.** Disease caused by mutation of the gene encoding fibrillin

_____ **16.** Reversible head deformity caused by birth-trauma

_____ **17.** A group of hereditary collagen disorders characterized by hyperelasticity and fragility of skin, joint hypermobility, frequent occurrence of hernias and even rupture of the arteries and viscera

_____ **18.** Transplacental IgG-mediated hemolytic reaction due to maternal-fetal blood group incompatibility

_____ **19.** The most common autosomal dominant tumor syndrome, characterized by the occurrence of multiple peripheral nerve tumors, cutaneous hyperpigmented macules (*café au lait* spots) and an increased risk for developing meningiomas and pheochromocytomas

_____ **20.** Mental retardation associated with trisomy of chromosome 21

Answers

1. **The answer is M.** A 47,XXY karotype is diagnostic of *Klinefelter syndrome.* The affected persons are phenotypically males, who exhibit eunuchoid body proportions in adolescence and never become fully masculinized. They have testicles devoid of germ cells and are, therefore, infertile. Serum FSH becomes elevated in these men at puberty. Typical male secondary features, such as pubic and chest hair do not develop unless the patients are treated with testosterone. The infertility cannot be cured.

2. **The answer is T.** A 45,X karotype is diagnostic of *Turner syndrome.* Typically these women exhibit short stature, webbing of the neck, and a broad chest. Their ovaries become depleted of oocytes early in life and transform into "streak gonads" composed predominantly of fibrous tissue. Because streak gonads do not respond to gonadotropins, Turner syndrome patients never experience puberty and suffer from primary amenorrhea. The internal and external genital organs form normally but are hypoplastic owing to inadequate estrogenic stimulation.

3. **The answer is K.** *Fragile-X syndrome* is a form of mental deficiency associated with increased fragility of the X-chromosome. The fragile site on the long arm of chromosome X contains multiple copies of the CCG triple nucleotide sequence. Approximately 80% of affected men have enlarged testicles.

4. **The answer is L.** Spontaneous hemarthrosis (bleeding into the joint cavity) is a typical feature of *hemophilia,* a sex-linked Mendelian disease, almost exclusively affecting males. The disease is caused by abnormalities of the genes encoding either coagulation factor VIII or IX, both of which are located on the X chromosome.

5. **The answer is A.** *Achondroplasia* is an autosomal dominant form of dwarfism caused by a disruption of endochondral ossification of large bones. The arms and legs of achondroplastic dwarfs are overly short in proportion to the head and body.

6. **The answer is P.** Multiple fractures of fetal bones in utero are a sign of severe *osteogenesis imperfecta* (OI), or a group of diseases related to mutations of the gene encoding collagen type I. Collagen type I is the major structural protein of bones and connective tissues found in all organs of the body. Bones lacking normal collagen type I are brittle and prone to fracturing. Sclerae lacking normal collagen type I reflect light differently from normal areas and thus appears bluish. Intrauterine fractures are features of type II and type III OI. Most cases of type III OI are stillborn.

7. **The answer is E.** Meconium ileus is a neonatal complication of *cystic fibrosis,* an autosomal recessive disease caused by mutations in the gene termed cystic fibrosis transmembrane conductance regulator (CFTR). Affected patients secrete highly viscous mucus into the lumen of many organs, notably the bronchi and pancreatic ducts. Meconium in fetal intestine may have an unusually firm consistency. Such material can obstruct the intestines, causing meconium ileus. Rupture of the intestines may spread the intestinal contents throughout the abdominal cavity (meconium peritonitis).

8. **The answer is J.** *Familial hypercholesterolemia* is an autosomal dominant disorder caused by mutations of the gene encoding the LDL receptor. It is one of the most common autosomal dominant disorders, affecting one in 500 adults in the United States. The gene defect affects the uptake of LDL in the liver, causing hypercholesterolemia. Clinically, the disease presents as severe atherosclerosis, which usually becomes symptomatic at an early age.

9. **The answer is Q.** *Phenylketonuria* is an autosomal recessive disorder caused by a mutation of the gene encoding phenylalanine hydroxylase, an enzyme that mediates the oxidation of phenylalanine to tyrosine. Excess phenylalanine is converted to phenylketones, which are excreted in the urine-hence the name of the disease and the mousy odor of urine. Major derivatives of tyrosine, such as melanin and neurotransmitters such as dopamine are not formed in adequate amounts. These deficiencies account, in part, for the clinical symptoms, such as lack of pigment in skin and hair. Hyperphenylalaninemia causes irreversible brain damage, which can be avoided by placing the infant on a phenylalanine-deficient diet.

10. **The answer is R.** *Spina bifida* is a congenital defect in the closure of the spinal canal. Like other dysraphic disorders (anencephaly, meningocele, meningomyelocele) spina bifida is of polygenic origin.

11. **The answer is S.** *Tay-Sachs* disease is a lethal, autosomal recessive error of metabolism caused by a mutation of the gene encoding the alpha unit of hexosaminidase. Clinically, it presents as progressive mental deterioration and blindness ("amaurotic idiocy"). The disease is also known as GM_2 gangliosidosis, type I. The enzyme defect causes the accumulation of GM_2 ganglioside in cells of many organs, most prominently in the brain and retina.

12. **The answer is B.** *Anencephaly* is a severe dysraphic disorder that impedes the closure of the cranium and prevents the proper development of the brain. Most babies with anencephaly die in utero or soon after birth.

13. **The answer is G.** *Duchenne muscular dystrophy* is an X-linked mendelian disorder characterized by severe progressive muscle wasting. The first signs of muscle weakness appear in early childhood. By school age, most affected boys are wheelchair-bound and by the age of 20 years, most of them have died.

14. **The answer is D.** *Cleft palate* is a polygenic disorder caused by the incomplete fusion of fetal parts that contribute to the formation of the mouth. The disease is three times more common in boys than in girls.

15. **The answer is N.** *Marfan syndrome* is caused by a mutation of gene encoding fibrillin. This molecule is a connective tissue protein that forms a scaffold for elastic fibers. Marfan syndrome features weakness of the arteries, joints, and lens ligaments.

16. **The answer is C.** *Cephalohematoma* is a birth-related subperiosteal hemorrhage over one of the calvarial bones. In most cases the hematoma resolves spontaneously, leaving no consequences.

17. **The answer is H.** *Ehlers-Danlos* syndrome comprises a group of clinically and genetically heterogeneous diseases characterized by hyperelasticity of the skin ("cutis laxa"), laxity of joints and other symptoms indicative of a systemic connective tissue defect. The pathologic changes reflect various defects in the synthesis and assembly of collagens type I or type III.

18. **The answer is I.** *Erythroblastosis fetalis* is an antibody-mediated hemolytic disease that affects the fetus in utero. It is usually caused by transplacental passage of maternal antibodies to antigens expressed on fetal red blood cells. Previously, it is most often caused by anti-Rh$^-$ antibodies. However, most Rh$^-$ mothers are today given prophylactic anti-Rh antibodies, Rh based fetal-maternal incompatibility is rare and most cases of hemolytic disease of the fetus and the newborn are caused by maternal antibodies to A, B, O antigens. Low antigenic expression of the A, B, O antigens on fetal red blood cells accounts for the mildness of such hemolytic reactions.

19. **The answer is O.** *Neurofibromatosis*, type I (von Recklinghausen disease) is an autosomal dominant tumor syndrome affecting at least 100,000 people in the United States. It is caused by a mutation of neurofibromin, a tumor suppressor gene. Affected persons have numerous neurofibromas, but also develop other tumors, notably meningiomas and pheochromocytomas.

20. **The answer is F.** *Down syndrome* reflects trisomy of chromosome 21 and is characterized by mental retardation and typical facial features, such as slanted eyes, epicanthal folds, lack of a philtrum, and macroglossia. Affected persons develop Alzheimer-like changes in the brain, usually by the age of 30-40 years. This is much earlier than in usual Alzheimer disease, which is a disorder of older ages.

Chapter 7

Hemodynamic Disorders

Questions

DIRECTIONS: Match each numbered statement with the most appropriate lettered item. Each lettered item can be used once, more than once, or not at all.

Hemodynamic Disorders

A. Active hyperemia
B. Anasarca
C. Ascites
D. Chronic passive congestion
E. Disseminated intravascular coagulation
F. Ecchymosis
G. Epistaxis
H. Fat embolism
I. Hemarthrosis
J. Hematemesis
K. Hematuria
L. Hematocephalus
M. Hematochezia
N. Hematoma
O. Hemoptysis
P. Melena
Q. Menorrhagia
R. Metrorrhagia
S. Purpura
T. Thromboembolism

_____ 1. Common symptom of acute cystitis

_____ 2. A common crippling feature of hemophilia

_____ 3. Complication of myocardial infarction that may cause a stroke

_____ 4. Characterized by multiple, dot-sized hemorrhages in the brain 3–5 days following fracture of the humerus

_____ 5. Common symptom of cavitary pulmonary tuberculosis

_____ 6. Black stools in a patient with a chronic bleeding duodenal ulcer

_____ 7. Complication of nose-picking

_____ 8. A potentially lethal complication of cirrhosis

_____ 9. Confluent skin hemorrhages around the eye ("black eye")

_____ 10. Accounts for the abdominal swelling in patients with cirrhosis

_____ 11. Generalized edema in a baby born with maternal-fetal Rh incompatibility

_____ 12. Feature of the nephrotic syndrome

_____ 13. Symptom of thrombocytopenia

_____ 14. Symptom of hypersensitivity vasculitis involving small blood vessels of the skin

_____ 15. Associated with septic shock, multiple organ failure, and microthrombi in capillaries, arterioles, and venules

_____ 16. Typical symptom of rectal carcinoma

_____ 17. Central nervous system complication of the neonatal respiratory distress syndrome in prematurely born infants

_____ 18. May be symptom of septic abortion

_____ 19. Heavy vaginal bleeding every 4 weeks in a 40-year-old woman, lasting 4–5 days

_____ 20. Blushing in a shy person

_____ 21. Associated with hemosiderin-laden macrophages (heart failure cells) in lungs of patients with left ventricular failure

Answers

1. **The answer is K.** *Hematuria* (blood in urine) is the most common symptom of cystitis. The bleeding stems from congested capillaries in the wall of the inflamed urinary bladder.

2. **The answer is I.** *Hemarthrosis* refers to bleeding into the joint cavity. It is associated with joint swelling and is a crippling complication of hemophilia. Repeated bleeding may cause deformities and may limit the mobility of the joints.

3. **The answer is T.** Mural thrombi overlying left ventricular infarcts are a source of arterial *thromboemboli*. Such emboli may occlude cerebral arteries and cause cerebral infarcts, known clinically as strokes.

4. **The answer is H.** *Fat emboli* originate from adipose tissue in the medulla of fractured long bones (e.g. femur or humerus). Fat carried by venous blood reaches the lungs, filters through the pulmonary circulation, enters arterial blood, and is disseminated throughout the body. The occlusion of cerebral capillaries is accompanied by petechial hemorrhages and is the most important complication of fat embolism.

5. **The answer is O.** *Hemoptysis* describes expectoration of blood and is a symptom of tuberculosis. However, it may accompany any other lung disease characterized by destruction of lung parenchyma. Massive bleeding stems from ruptured pulmonary arteries and veins.

6. **The answer is P.** *Melena* (black stool) is a symptom of upper gastrointestinal bleeding. Blood from ruptured esophageal varices, gastritis, or

peptic ulcer is partially digested by hydrochloric acid. Hemoglobin is transformed into a black pigment (hematin), which imparts the typical coffee-grounds color to the stool.

7. **The answer is G.** *Epistaxis* is the term used for nosebleed, which is most often caused mechanically (e.g., nose-picking or a punch to the nose).

8. **The answer is J.** *Hematemesis* (bloody vomit) often originates from ruptured esophageal varices and is a potentially lethal complication of cirrhosis.

9. **The answer is S.** "Black eye" represents a confluent superficial skin hemorrhage and is an example of *ecchymosis*.

10. **The answer is C.** A protruding belly in patients with cirrhosis is caused by *ascites* (i.e., accumulation of serous fluid in the abdominal cavity). It is primarily a consequence of portal hypertension and hypoalbuminemia, which are common complications of cirrhosis.

11. **The answer is B.** Maternal/fetal Rh incompatibility occurs when the fetus is Rh$^+$ and the mother is sensitized to Rh$^+$ antigen (IgG antibodies to Rh$^+$ fetal erythrocytes). The condition may result in severe hydrops fetus. Generalized edema is called *anasarca* and is caused by intravascular hemolysis of fetal red blood cells. The resulting anemia strains the fetal heart, which finally fails. Anasarca is thus a consequence of fetal heart failure.

12. **The answer is B.** Generalized edema *(anasarca)* develops in nephrotic syndrome, owing to hypoproteinemia caused by the loss of protein in urine.

13. **The answer is S.** *Purpura* refers to widespread capillary bleeding, which is typical of thrombocytopenia. Similar pin-point hemorrhages, which may become confluent, are also seen in conditions that affect small blood vessels, capillaries, and venules (e.g., Henoch-Schönlein purpura or vitamin C deficiency).

14. **The answer is S.** *Purpura* is a symptom of hypersensitivity vasculitis, a disease that presents with leukocytoclastic inflammation of dermal venules.

15. **The answer is E.** *Disseminated intravascular coagulation* (DIC) is a thrombotic microangiopathy, which typically occurs in septic shock. Fibrin thrombi form in small blood vessels because of uncontrollable coagulopathy, which consumes fibrin and other coagulation factors. Once the coagulation factors are depleted from the circulating blood, uncontrollable hemorrhage ensues.

16. **The answer is M.** *Hematochezia* (i.e., rectal bleeding) is a symptom of rectal cancer.

17. **The answer is L.** *Hematocephalus* refers to bleeding into the lateral ventricles of the brain and is a complication of neonatal respiratory distress syndrome. Pulmonary lesions, such as atelectasis and hyaline membranes, typically develop in this syndrome, leading to anoxia of the brain. As a result, hemorrhages into the periventricular germinal matrix occur and spread into the cerebral ventricles.

18. **The answer is R.** *Metrorrhagia* is the term for severe vaginal hemorrhage and is one of the complications of septic abortion. Similar hemorrhages

of uterine origin may follow therapeutic abortion or may be a symptom of endometrial cancer or hyperplasia.

19. **The answer is Q.** *Menorrhagia* represents heavy menstrual bleeding. It occurs at intervals typical of the regular menstrual cycle, in contrast to metrorrhagia, which is unrelated to the cycle.

20. **The answer is A.** Blushing results from *active hyperemia* caused by neurogenic relaxation of the precapillary sphincters in the facial arterioles.

21. **The answer is D.** Left ventricular failure leads to *chronic passive congestion* of the lungs. Blood leaks from the congested pulmonary capillaries into the alveoli. Alveolar macrophages degrade red blood cells and accumulate hemosiderin, which is derived from partially digested hemoglobin. These hemosiderin-laden macrophages are called "heart failure cells" and are typically found in the alveoli but may be also expectorated in the sputum.

Chapter 8

Environmental and Nutritional Pathology

Questions

DIRECTIONS: Match each numbered statement with the most appropriate lettered item. Each lettered item can be used once, more than once, or not at all.

Minerals

A. Arsenic
B. Barium
C. Cadmium
D. Copper
E. Iron
F. Lead
G. Mercury
H. Nickel
I. Zinc

_____ 1. Metaphyseal densities in growing bones

_____ 2. Peripheral motor neuropathy in adults and encephalopathy in children

_____ 3. Anemia with basophilic stippling of erythrocytes

_____ 4. Fanconi syndrome and inclusion bodies in the nuclei of proximal tubular cells in the kidney

_____ 5. Inorganic metal compounds predominantly affect the kidney and the organic compounds injure the brain

_____ 6. Minamata disease

_____ 7. Chronic environmental exposure causes cancer of the skin and upper respiratory tract

_____ 8. Fumes cause acute pulmonary edema

_____ 9. Hypersensitivity dermatitis caused by costume jewelry

_____ 10. Chronic exposure may cause cancer of the nasal cavity

Physical and Thermal Injury

A. Abrasion
B. Bullet wound
C. Burns
D. Commotion
E. Contusion
F. Electrical injury
G. Frostbite
H. Laceration
I. Trench foot

_____ **11.** Causes crystallization of intracellular water

_____ **12.** Caused by prolonged immersion in cold water

_____ **13.** Hemoconcentration may occur in severe injury

_____ **14.** Ventricular fibrillation is a common cause of instantaneous death

_____ **15.** Bullae develop rapidly

_____ **16.** Round hole on the skin surface

_____ **17.** Skin hole with ragged edges

_____ **18.** Tear of tissues caused by tangential impact

_____ **19.** Superficial skin defect caused by tangential impact

_____ **20.** "Black eye"

Radiation Injury

A. Localized radiation treatment of cancer
B. Acute total-body radiation, 300 rad
C. Acute total-body radiation, 1000 rad
D. Acute total-body radiation, 2000 rad
E. Survivors of atomic bomb explosions

_____ **21.** Hematopoietic failure after 2 weeks

_____ **22.** Death due to gastrointestinal syndrome within 3 days

_____ **23.** Central nervous system symptoms within hours

_____ **24.** Fibrosing pneumonitis

_____ **25.** Radiodermatitis

_____ **26.** Leukemia

Vitamin Deficiencies

A. A
B. B_1 (thiamine)
C. B_2 (riboflavin)
D. B_{12}
E. C
F. D
G. E
H. Folic acid

    I. K

    J. Niacin

    K. Pyridoxine

_____ **27.** Dermatitis, diarrhea, and dementia

_____ **28.** Heart failure

_____ **29.** Xerophthalmia

_____ **30.** Cheilosis

_____ **31.** Demyelination of anterior columns

_____ **32.** Anemia caused by atrophic gastritis

_____ **33.** Megaloblastic anemia secondary to antineoplastic or antiepileptic drug treatment

_____ **34.** Pregnancy-related anemia

_____ **35.** Celiac disease associated with megaloblastic anemia

_____ **36.** Megaloblastic anemia of Crohn disease

_____ **37.** Poor wound healing and perifollicular petechiae in the skin

_____ **38.** Rickets

Answers

1. **The answer is F.** *Lead* is deposited in the metaphysis of growing bones. These "lead lines" are detected radiologically and are important signs of pica-related, chronic lead toxicity in children.

2. **The answer is F.** *Lead* toxicity primarily affects three major organ systems: the nervous system, the kidneys, and the hemopoietic system. In children the neurologic symptoms (encephalopathy) are more prominent, whereas in adults peripheral neuropathy is more conspicuous.

3. **The answer is F.** *Lead* inhibits delta-aminolevulinic acid dehydratase and ferrochelatase (enzymes essential for heme synthesis) thereby causing microcytic hypochromic anemia. The inhibition of heme synthesis leads to basophilic stippling of erythrocytes, which is due to residual ribosome clusters in the cytoplasm.

4. **The answer is F.** *Lead* injures the proximal renal tubules and is recognized morphologically by intranuclear lead inclusions. Aminoaciduria, glycosuria, and phosphaturia (Fanconi syndrome) are the functional counterparts.

5. **The answer is G.** Inorganic *mercury* predominantly affects the kidneys, whereas the organic form acts mostly on the central nervous system. The toxic effects of mercury on the brain present as tremor, confusion, and various mental symptoms.

6. **The answer is G.** "Minamata disease" refers to the severe neurotoxicity that was caused by *mercury* poisoning from the consumption of contaminated fish in the Minamata Bay in Japan. It presents with a variety of central and peripheral nerve symptoms, including visual and hearing impairment, tremor, lack of motor coordination, paresthesias, and mental dysfunction.

7. **The answer is A.** *Arsenic* is an environmental carcinogen unequivocally linked to human cancer. Arsenic-related cancers among industrial vineyard workers arise in the skin and upper respiratory tract.

8. **The answer is C.** *Cadmium* fumes are extremely toxic and cause massive pulmonary edema. The kidney may also be injured, since cadmium is excreted in urine.

9. **The answer is H.** *Nickel* in coins or costume jewelry may cause a delayed hypersensitivity reaction and chronic dermatitis.

10. **The answer is H.** Workers in the *nickel* industry and nickel mines have shown an increased incidence of cancer of the lung and the entire respiratory tract, most prominently in the nasal sinuses.

11. **The answer is G.** *Frostbite* is caused by severe hypothermia and is marked by crystallization of intracellular water.

12. **The answer is I.** Trenchfoot is caused by prolonged immersion in cold water. The temperature is not low enough to freeze the tissue, but nevertheless causes cell damage.

13. **The answer is C.** Massive cutaneous burns result in a fluid loss, which may amount to 0.3 ml/cm^2 of body surface. This "empties" the interstitial fluid compartments and causes a shift of fluid from the circulation into the interstitium. Total blood volume is reduced, resulting in hemoconcentration.

14. **The answer is F.** *Electrical injury* induces disturbances in the conduction of impulses in the heart, and rapid death may occur as a result of ventricular fibrillation.

15. **The answer is C.** Bullae (i.e., fluid-filled spaces in the epidermis) are secondary to *burn-related* necrosis of basal cells in the epidermis and the separation of the dermis from the epidermis. The fluid is a transudate of interstitial fluid and plasma.

16. **The answer is B.** A typical entrance wound caused by a fast-moving *bullet* is round.

17. **The answer is B.** The exit *bullet wound* has ragged edges, reflecting the combined impact of the bullet and particles of clothes and tissue carried along with it.

18. **The answer is H.** A *laceration* is a tissue tear produced by a tangential force that causes unidirectional displacement of different components of the affected body part.

19. **The answer is A.** An *abrasion* results from a tangential impact that crushes the surface of the skin, thereby causing a superficial defect in the epidermis. Abraded lacerations exhibit both tears and surface defects.

20. **The answer is E.** A "black eye" is a typical example of a *contusion* caused by a localized mechanical injury that leads to tissue damage and hemorrhage.

21. **The answer is B.** Acute total-body *irradiation of about 300 rad* causes depression of the bone marrow, and symptoms of granulocytopenia and thrombocytopenia develop within 2 weeks. Anemia follows more slowly, because the red blood cells live longer than leukocytes and platelets.

22. The answer is C. A *radiation dose of about 1000 rad* causes destruction of tissues composed of proliferating cells. Damage to the gastrointestinal tract is the most serious consequence and ensues within days of exposure. Death results from massive fluid loss from the denuded intestinal mucosa and superimposed infection.

23. The answer is D. *Radiation doses of 2000 rad* or higher cause death within hours as a result of cerebral edema and neuronal necrosis.

24. The answer is A. *Localized radiation* therapy for cancer produces fibrosing lesions in the lungs, intestine, pericardium, and many other sites.

25. The answer is A. Radiodermatitis is characterized by atrophy of the epidermis, hyperkeratosis, hyperpigmentation, and telangiectatic dilatation of small blood vessels in the dermis. It is the most common consequence of *localized radiation* therapy.

26. The answer is E. The survivors of the *atomic bomb blasts* in Japan suffered an increased incidence of acute nonlymphocytic leukemia. The incidence of chronic myelogenous leukemia also was increased, and there were more solid tissue tumors, primarily cancers of the breast, lung, and thyroid.

27. The answer is J. The three D's—dermatitis, diarrhea, and dementia—are features of *niacin* deficiency, commonly termed "pellagra." Severe pellagra adds another D—death.

28. The answer is B. In so-called wet beri-beri, which reflects *thiamine* deficiency, heart failure and edema predominate over polyneuropathy, which is the dominant feature of "dry beri-beri."

29. The answer is A. *Vitamin A* deficiency causes squamous metaplasia at a number of sites. In the cornea it leads to xerophthalmia (dry eye), which may progress to softening of the tissue (keratomalacia).

30. The answer is C. Cheilosis refers to fissures at the angles of the mouth and is a common finding in B_2 *riboflavin* deficiency.

31. The answer is D. Spinal cord lesions occur in *vitamin B_{12}* deficiency, but not in folic acid deficiency.

32. The answer is D. Patients with atrophic gastritis lack the intrinsic factor needed for the absorption of *vitamin B_{12}.* Since intrinsic factor is essential for B_{12} vitamin absorption, patients with atrophic gastritis develop vitamin B_{12} deficiency and therefore megaloblastic anemia (pernicious anemia).

33. The answer is H. Various folate antagonists used in cancer chemotherapy compete with *folic acid* and cause symptoms of folic acid deficiency. Similar symptoms may be caused by certain drugs (e.g., the antiepileptic agent diphenyl hydantoin, which interfere with the absorption of folic acid in the intestine).

34. The answer is H. It has been estimated that two-thirds of anemic pregnant women are *folate*-deficient.

35. The answer is H. *Folic acid* is absorbed in the upper third of the small intestine; therefore, celiac disease may be associated with folate deficiency.

36. The answer is D. *Vitamin B_{12}* is absorbed in the terminal ileum. Hence a deficiency of this vitamin may occur in Crohn disease ("terminal ileitis").

37. **The answer is E.** *Vitamin C* is essential for collagen synthesis, and its deficiency results in poor wound healing. Perifollicular hemorrhages arise from capillaries that have weak walls and are easily damaged by minor trauma.

38. **The answer is F.** Rickets is the syndrome caused by *vitamin D* deficiency in growing children. In adults, the equivalent syndrome is termed *osteomalacia*.

Chapter 9

Infectious and Parasitic Diseases

DIRECTIONS: Choose the one best answer.

_____ 1. The purification of drinking water and better hygiene in the United States have decreased the incidence of
A. tuberculosis.
B. smallpox.
C. hepatitis A.
D. pertussis.
E. malaria.

_____ 2. Koch's postulates include all the following *except*
A. the causative organism is present in all examples of the disease.
B. the causative organism can be recovered in pure form from the lesions.
C. the isolated organism produces the disease in experimental animals.
D. the organism can be recovered from the lesions of the animal.
E. the animal can be cured with the same drug that cures the disease in humans.

_____ 3. The characteristic pathologic changes in yellow fever are in the
A. brain.
B. lung.
C. liver.
D. spleen.
E. stomach.

_____ 4. Which of the following statements is true for poliomyelitis?
A. The infection is transmitted by animal vectors.
B. The virus enters the body through the upper respiratory tract.
C. The virus reaches the central nervous system by migrating along peripheral nerves.
D. The anterior horn cells of the spinal cord are the principal site of injury.
E. A vigorous T cell response prevents the disease.

_____ **5.** Which of the following statements is true for smallpox?
   A. Still a major health problem in underdeveloped countries.
   B. Transmitted by fecal/oral route.
   C. Causes multiloculated vesicles owing to degeneration of epidermal cells.
   D. Jaundice is a prominent feature.
   E. The disease exacerbates endogenous viruses, which then cause major complications.

_____ **6.** The typical histologic feature common to herpes simplex infection and varicella (chicken pox) is the formation of
   A. acidophilic bodies.
   B. intranuclear inclusions.
   C. granulomas with giant cells.
   D. plasma cell response.
   E. eosinophilia.

_____ **7.** Persons infected with herpes simplex virus type 2 (genital herpes) harbor the virus in a latent form in the
   A. mucosa of the external genitalia.
   B. epithelial cells of the internal genital organs.
   C. germ cells.
   D. connective tissue of the penis or vagina.
   E. sacral ganglia.

_____ **8.** All the following are true for cytomegalovirus *except*
   A. most adults are seropositive.
   B. it may be transmitted transplacentally.
   C. most congenital infections produce no symptoms.
   D. in AIDS patients it most often causes encephalitis.
   E. infected cells appear enlarged.

_____ **9.** The atypical lymphoid cells in the peripheral blood of patients with infectious mononucleosis are
   A. infected with Epstein-Barr virus.
   B. B cell precursors.
   C. activated mature B cells.
   D. activated T cells.
   E. monocytes.

_____ **10.** A complication of infectious mononucleosis is
   A. Burkitt lymphoma.
   B. cerebral abscess.
   C. rupture of the spleen.
   D. cirrhosis of the liver.
   E. gonadal atrophy.

_____ **11.** A rash beginning in the form of pink papules behind the ears that quickly becomes maculopapular and spreads over the face and down the neck, trunk, and limbs is typical of
   A. mumps.
   B. measles (rubeola).
   C. varicella.
   D. infectious mononucleosis.
   E. rotavirus infection.

_____ **12.** The lungs of a child who died of acute pneumonia showed numerous Warthin-Finkeldey giant cells with up to 100 nuclei. This child had an infection caused by

   A. Epstein-Barr virus.
   B. cytomegalovirus.
   C. measles virus.
   D. rubellavirus.
   E. mumps virus.

_____ **13.** Necrotizing bronchitis and diffuse hemorrhagic necrotizing pneumonia of adults, occasionally seen in epidemic form, is caused by

   A. influenza virus A.
   B. rhinovirus.
   C. respiratory syncytial virus.
   D. rotavirus.
   E. Norwalk-like viruses.

_____ **14.** Interstitial pneumonia is caused by infection with all the following agents *except*

   A. adenovirus.
   B. orthomyxoviruses.
   C. *Mycoplasma pneumoniae.*
   D. *Chlamydia psittaci.*
   E. *Streptococcus pneumoniae.*

_____ **15.** Ocular lesions caused by *Chlamydia trachomatis* include all the following *except*

   A. hyperemia of the conjunctiva.
   B. pannus formation.
   C. lymphocytic infiltrates.
   D. scarring.
   E. retinal ablation.

_____ **16.** Lymphogranuloma venereum typically presents with all the following *except*

   A. pustular or vesicular lesions on the penis or vagina.
   B. lymphadenopathy.
   C. coalescing abscesses surrounded by a zone of palisaded epithelioid cells.
   D. proctitis in homosexuals.
   E. urethritis.

_____ **17.** Epidemic typhus is characterized by all the following *except*

   A. Rickettsiae in endothelial cells.
   B. fibrin thrombi in small blood vessels.
   C. vasculitis.
   D. typhus nodules composed of mononuclear cells.
   E. abscesses.

_____ **18.** Vasculitis is found in all the following rickettsial infections *except*

   A. epidemic typhus (louseborne).
   B. endemic (murine) typhus.
   C. Rocky Mountain spotted fever.
   D. scrub typhus (tsutsugamushi disease).
   E. Q fever.

_____ **19.** Which of the following lesions is found in all stages of syphilis?

    A. Chancre
    B. Condylomata lata
    C. Gummas
    D. Vasculitis
    E. Tabes dorsalis

_____ **20.** Charcot joint (i.e., degenerative arthritis of tertiary syphilis) is a consequence of

    A. immune complex formation.
    B. central paresis.
    C. gumma in the synovium.
    D. severe vasculitis in the synovium.
    E. tabes dorsalis.

_____ **21.** More than 90% of all patients with anthrax have

    A. gastrointestinal hemorrhages.
    B. septicemia.
    C. hemorrhagic pneumonia.
    D. skin lesions.
    E. mucosal ulcerations.

_____ **22.** During the phases of active invasion and bacteremia in typhoid fever, *Salmonella typhi* can be found in all the following organs *except*

    A. terminal ileum.
    B. mesenteric lymph nodes.
    C. liver.
    D. esophagus.
    E. blood.

_____ **23.** Infiltrates in the lungs caused by *Legionella pneumophila* usually contain

    A. macrophages.
    B. lymphocytes.
    C. basophils.
    D. eosinophils.
    E. plasma cells.

_____ **24.** Cholera is characterized by

    A. ulceration of the small intestinal mucosa.
    B. granulomas overlying Peyer's patches.
    C. crypt abscesses in the large intestine.
    D. severe watery diarrhea.
    E. peritonitis.

_____ **25.** Clostridium species may cause all the following *except*

    A. necrotizing enteritis.
    B. necrosis of skeletal muscle.
    C. generalized muscle spasm.
    D. paralysis of muscles innervated by cranial nerves.
    E. brain abscess.

_____ **26.** Which of the following is a typical complication of diphtherial infection?

A. Peritonitis
B. Meningitis
C. Myocarditis
D. Hepatitis
E. Nephritis

_____ **27.** Impetigo is caused by

A. *Clostridium difficile.*
B. *Staphylococcus aureus.*
C. *Corynebacterium diphtheriae.*
D. *Klebsiela pneumoniae.*
E. *Pseudomonas aeruginosa.*

_____ **28.** Which of the following is a noninfectious complication of strep-tococcal pharyngitis?

A. Rheumatoid arthritis
B. Acute glomerulonephritis
C. Meningitis
D. Hepatitis
E. Orchitis

_____ **29.** Which of the following is a potentially lethal complication of meningococcal infection?

A. Waterhouse-Friderichsen syndrome
B. Myocarditis
C. Hepatitis
D. Glomerulonephritis
E. Endometritis

_____ **30.** Acute gonococcal infection in women typically produces inflam-mation of the

A. vulva.
B. endocervix.
C. vagina.
D. ovary.
E. parametrium.

_____ **31.** Secondary pulmonary tuberculosis may be complicated by all the following *except*

A. scarring.
B. calcification.
C. massive hemorrhage.
D. pleurisy.
E. carcinoma.

_____ **32.** At autopsy, patients with fatal trypanosomiasis most commonly exhibit

A. meningoencephalitis.
B. massive necrosis of liver cells.
C. lung abscesses.
D. heart abscesses.
E. endocarditis.

INSTRUCTIONS: Match each numbered word or phrase with the most appropriate pathogen from the list of lettered answers. Each lettered item can be used once, more than once, or not at all.

A. *Ascaris lumbricoides*
B. *Aspergillus fumigatus*
C. *Candida albicans*
D. *Clonorchis sinensis*
E. *Cryptosporidium*
F. *Entamoeba histolytica*
G. *Giardia lamblia*
H. *Histoplasma capsulatum*
I. *Leishmania donovani*

J. *Naegleria fowleri*
K. *Plasmodium falciparum*
L. *Pneumocystis carinii*
M. *Schistosoma haematobium*
N. *Sporothrix schenkii*
O. *Strongyloides stercoralis*
P. *Toxoplasma gondii*
Q. *Trichinella spiralis*
R. *Trichophyton*

_____ **33.** Hemoglobinuric nephrosis

_____ **34.** Perivascular brain hemorrhages

_____ **35.** Liver and spleen enlarged by macrophages that contain live parasitic forms

_____ **36.** Darkening of the skin pancytopenia, bleeding tendency

_____ **37.** Transplacental infection of the fetus

_____ **38.** Cause of pneumonia in AIDS

_____ **39.** Cause of colonic ulcers

_____ **40.** Hepatic abscess

_____ **41.** Meningoencephalitis develops following acute rhinitis

_____ **42.** Cause of inflammation of terminal ileum and diarrhea in patients with AIDS

_____ **43.** Harmless commensal, but may cause intermittent diarrhea, especially in children

_____ **44.** Fungus ball in the lung

_____ **45.** Angiocentric lesions

_____ **46.** Oral thrush in children

_____ **47.** Ulcerated nodule with satellite nodules along the lymphatic drainage

_____ **48.** Pulmonary lesions similar to tuberculosis

_____ **49.** Superficial skin mycosis involving the hair

_____ **50.** Myositis

_____ **51.** Hyperinfection occurs in immunosuppressed persons

_____ **52.** Most common helminthic infection, although most often asymptomatic

_____ **53.** Bladder cancer

_____ **54.** Biliary infection

_____ **55.** Cholangiocarcinoma

Answers

1. **The answer is C.** *Hepatitis A* is transmitted by the oral route, and its incidence is still high in many countries with poor hygiene.

2. **The answer is E.** Koch's postulates deal with the identification, isolation, and experimental reproduction of infectious diseases. They are not concerned with the *response to therapy*.

3. **The answer is C.** The most characteristic lesions of yellow fever are in the *liver*, which shows typical midzonal necrosis of single hepatocytes, known as acidophilic or "Councilman" bodies. Jaundice is followed by renal failure and widespread hemorrhages.

4. **The answer is D.** Poliomyelitis is a water-borne infection transmitted through the fecal/oral route. The virus does not need vectors for completion of the cycle. Poliovirus enters the mucosa of the small intestine and then causes viremia. It does not reach the central nervous system along nerves. The *anterior horn cells of the spinal cord* are typically destroyed, causing a lower motor neuron type of paralysis.

5. **The answer is C.** Smallpox has now been eradicated by successful worldwide vaccination. Since the virus is stable (i.e., mutations do not occur often and there are no animal reservoirs), the virus is likely to remain eradicated. Previously, it was transmitted from infected individuals by respiratory droplets. The skin is the main site of viral replication. The virus causes degeneration of epidermal cells and the formation of *multilocular vesicles* and bullae. These may become infected with bacteria and heal by scarring. Ocular scars were a major cause of blindness. Smallpox does not affect the liver or activate endogenous viruses.

6. **The answer is B.** *Viral inclusions* are typically located in the *nucleus* in herpes and varicella infections. They can be seen by light microscopy and even better by electron microscopy. Both infections lead to necrosis of infected cells, but not in the form of acidophilic bodies. The latter are seen in the liver in viral hepatitis and yellow fever and represent necrotic single hepatocytes. Giant cells also occur in herpes infection, owing to the fusion of infected epithelial cells, but they are not part of granulomas.

7. **The answer is E.** Herpesvirus ascends from the genital lesions along the sensory neurons and survives in a latent form in the *sacral ganglia*. Nonspecific stimuli, including sexual intercourse and menses, reactivate the virus, which descends within the axons to the genital mucosa. It produces recurrent blisters on the external and internal genitalia.

8. **The answer is D.** As implied in the name, cytomegalovirus causes a marked enlargement of infected cells, which contain typical intranuclear and often cytoplasmic inclusions. The virus may be transmitted from mother to child transplacentally or during delivery (perinatal infection). Infected children are, however, usually asymptomatic. In adults, cytomegalovirus may be transmitted through close contact, sexual encounters, transfusions, transplantation, and even the inhalation of infected particles. In symptomatic infants and children, central nervous symptoms predominate, in contrast to adults, in whom the virus produces mostly respiratory and gastrointestinal symptoms; it does not cause *encephalitis* in adults.

9. **The answer is D.** Epstein-Barr virus, a herpesvirus that causes infectious mononucleosis, infects B-lymphocytes. In response to virus-induced changes in the B-lymphocytes, T cells are activated. *Activated T cells* appear in the peripheral blood as so-called atypical lymphocytes. The blood shows lymphocytosis and monocytosis, and anemia and thrombocytopenia are common.

10. **The answer is C.** Splenomegaly often develops in infectious mononucleosis because of hyperplasia of lymphoid tissue, infiltration of the spleen with lymphoid cells, and edema. Such an enlarged *spleen may rupture* easily after minor trauma, and patients should therefore be advised to avoid contact sports. Burkitt lymphoma is pathogenetically related to the Epstein-Barr virus (EBV), but its exact role is not known. EBV infection is common worldwide, whereas Burkitt lymphoma is endemic to sub-Saharan Africa. Viral encephalitis, but not brain abscess, occurs in infectious mononucleosis, albeit rarely. Although hepatitis is common, and liver function tests are often abnormal, cirrhosis does not develop. Likewise, gonadal atrophy is not a complication of EBV infection.

11. **The answer is B.** *Measles* is an exanthematous disease characterized by a centrifugal rash.

12. **The answer is C.** Warthin-Finkeldey giant cells are pathognomonic of *measles* infection. The atypical lymphoid cells and immunoblasts characteristic of infection with Epstein-Barr virus are not multinucleated. Cytomegalovirus-infected cells are very large and contain nuclear and possibly cytoplasmic viral inclusions, but they are not multinucleated. Rubella and mumps viruses induce a mononuclear infiltrate composed of lymphocytes, macrophages, and plasma cells, but no giant cells.

13. **The answer is A.** *Influenza A* is the most common cause of viral pneumonia in adults and is the only influenza virus that causes epidemics and pandemics. Rhinovirus is the most frequent cause of the "common cold." Rotavirus and Norwalk-like agents are causes of diarrhea in children. Rotavirus is the most common cause of childhood diarrhea in developed countries.

14. **The answer is E.** Adenoviruses, especially those belonging to subgroup B, are a common cause of viral pneumonia in young children and in army recruits. Orthomyxoviruses cause influenza and pneumonia as a common extension of upper respiratory tract infection. *Mycoplasma pneumoniae* is a slowly growing microorganism, larger than most viruses but smaller than bacteria, which can replicate outside the cells. These microorganisms cause "atypical pneumonia," mostly in children and young adults, especially those living in close contact. *Chlamydia psittaci* is the cause of respiratory psittacosis, usually spread by close contact with birds and their excreta. All these microorganisms cause interstitial, rather than exudative, alveolar pneumonia. *Streptococal pneumonia* causes an intraalveolar exudate, thereby producing either lobar or lobular pneumonia (bronchopneumonia).

15. **The answer is E.** *Chlamydia trachomatis* produces an acute and chronic inflammation of the conjunctiva and cornea called *trachoma.* In some patients there is a prominent vascular granulation tissue (pannus), which contains lymphoid infiltrates and leads to scarring. Infected epithelial cells contain diagnostic intracytoplasmic bodies. *The retina is not affected.*

16. **The answer is E.** Genital infections in lymphogranuloma venereum usually resolve completely, even without adequate therapy. Chronic ulcers, such as vulvar esthiomene, occur only rarely. Vesicular lesions on the genitalia are typically accompanied by enlarged lymph nodes, which contain confluent abscesses rimmed by epithelioid cells. These have the appearance of granulomas and are similar to those seen in cat scratch disease. Anal intercourse may transmit the infection and cause proctocolitis. *Urethritis* typical of gonorrhea or chylamidial infections is not found.

17. **The answer is E.** *Rickettsia prowazekii* multiplies in and injures the endothelial cells of blood vessels. Thrombi form inside small blood vessels, owing to the damage to the endothelial lining. Bleeding occurs through the inflamed and disrupted walls of small blood vessels. The aggregates of lymphocytes, macrophages, and plasma cells surrounding the infected blood vessels form so-called typhus nodules. *Abscesses* are not found.

18. **The answer is E.** All rickettsial infections except for *Q fever* are characterized by the invasion of endothelial cells by microorganisms and subsequent vasculitis. By contrast, Q fever features granulomas.

19. **The answer is D.** Syphilitic *vasculitis*, characterized by infiltrates of lymphocytes and plasma cells around small blood vessels, occurs in all stages of syphilis. The chancre is typical of primary syphilis. Condyloma latum is a skin and mucosal lesion of secondary syphilis. Gummas and tabes dorsalis are typical of tertiary syphilis.

20. **The answer is E.** Degeneration of large joints (Charcot joints) is a consequence of *tabes dorsalis*. The latter reflects the destruction of dorsal spiral columns and afferent pathways that are essential for normal coordinated movements of the extremities. Owing to this neurologic disease, the joints are exposed to undue stress, causing degeneration of articular cartilage and deformities of the joint.

21. **The answer is D.** *Bacillus anthracis* enters the body, in more than 95% of cases, through small breaks in the *skin*. The organism causes local hemorrhagic pustules, which may progress to carbuncles. These are typically black, because of the extravasation of blood. The name of the disease derives from the Greek word for coal (anthrax). Respiratory infection, acquired from spores inhaled from contaminated raw wool (wool sorters disease), is much less common. Anthrax may be complicated by septicemia, but this is uncommon. Also rare is gastrointestinal infection, which may cause hemorrhagic ulcers in the stomach.

22. **The answer is D.** Following ingestion, *Salmonella typhi* passes through the upper gastrointestinal tract. The organisms that survive gastric acidity attach to the surface of the small intestine, from which they enter the lymphatics and the blood. *S. typhi* is sequestered by phagocytic cells in the liver, lymph nodes, spleen, and bone marrow. In addition to the intestinal lesions, the infection causes enlargement of mesenteric lymph nodes, splenomegaly, and hepatomegaly. *The esophagus is not affected.*

23. **The answer is A.** Legionella infection primarily evokes a *macrophage* response. Macrophages are seen in early pulmonary lesions and usually contain phagocytosed organisms. The subsequent necrosis of lung tissue attracts neutrophils, but lymphocytes, basophils, and plasma cells are not seen.

24. **The answer is D.** Cholera, caused by *Vibrio cholerae*, is basically an infection limited to the lumen of the small intestine. The bacteria secrete an enterotoxin that causes *watery diarrhea*. The mucosa of the intestine does not show any significant pathologic changes.

25. **The answer is E.** Food poisoning and necrotizing enteritis are caused by the enterotoxins of *C. perfringens*. *C. perfringens* type A is the most common cause of gas gangrene following wound infection or septic abortion. *C. tetani* produces a potent neurotoxin that causes tetany and generalized muscle spasms, which are often fatal. By contrast, *C. botulinum* neurotoxin causes paralysis, prominently but not exclusively, involving the cranial nerves. *Clostridia do not cause brain abscesses.*

26. **The answer is C.** Diphtheria typically begins as a pseudomembranous pharyngitis. Diphtheria exotoxin causes necrosis of epithelial cells on the mucosal surface, exudation of fibrin, and the accumulation of polymorphonuclear leukocytes. Together with necrotic cell debris, these form the pseudomembranes. Exotoxin absorbed into the circulation causes necrosis of *cardiac myocytes*, usually followed by infiltration of the heart by scavenger macrophages. Diphtheria exotoxin also causes demyelinating injury of the peripheral nerves. Other major organs such as the liver are not affected, and if the patient survives, the initial injury is not followed by permanent complications.

27. **The answer is B.** Three species of *Staphylococcus* are pathogenic in humans. These may be coagulase-positive, such as *S. aureus*, or coagulase-negative, such as *S. epidermidis* and *S. saprophyticus*. The latter two were formerly called *S. albus* because they form white, rather than yellow, colonies on blood agar. Most purulent infections are caused by *S. aureus*.

28. **The answer is B.** Acute poststreptococcal *glomerulonephritis* is caused by immune complexes, but the antigen has not been identified. Rheumatoid arthritis is not related to streptococcal infection, in contrast to rheumatic fever. Meningitis results from meningeal seeding of bacteria following pneumonia or sepsis caused by streptococci, especially *S. pneumoniae*.

29. **The answer is A.** Meningococcal sepsis is marked by profound endotoxemic shock and disseminated intravascular coagulation, known as *"Waterhouse-Friderichsen syndrome."* Acute meningococcal meningitis may develop very rapidly and is often fatal.

30. **The answer is B.** The squamous epithelium of the vagina and the vulva is relatively resistant to gonococcal invasion, in contrast to the transitional epithelium of the urethra and the columnar epithelium of the *endocervix*. In later stages, the infection may spread to the fallopian tubes and cause PID.

31. **The answer is E.** The lesions of secondary tuberculosis often cavitate or become fibrotic. The healed secondary lesion frequently exhibits dystrophic calcification. Erosion of blood vessels by tuberculous lesions may be the cause of bleeding from large pulmonary blood vessels. The lesions of secondary tuberculosis may involve the pleura, causing pleurisy and fluid accumulation in the pleural cavity. *Tuberculosis does not cause cancer.*

32. **The answer is A.** Death in trypanosomiasis is typically caused by *meningoencephalitis*, marked by perivascular infiltrates of lymphocytes and plasma cells. Lymphoid hyperplasia and lymphoid infiltrates may be widespread and involve all organs, including the heart. Trypanosomes are difficult to find in tissue sections.

33. **The answer is K.** Hemoglobinuric nephrosis in *Falciparum malaria* is caused by massive intravascular hemolysis.

34. **The answer is K.** In malaria, capillaries of the brain are especially prone to occlusion by parasitized erythrocytes, with subsequent *perivascular hemorrhages* and microinfarcts.

35. **The answer is I.** In *leishmaniasis*, the spleen, liver, and bone marrow contain innumerable foamy macrophages that contain amastigotes of *L. donovani*.

36. **The answer is I.** Visceral *leishmaniasis*, also known as "Kala azar" (Hindi, meaning "black fever"), is associated with darkening of the skin. Pancytopenia develops and may predispose to uncontrollable bleeding or bacterial superinfection.

37. **The answer is P.** *Toxoplasmosis* may be transmitted to the fetus transplacentally, even when the mother is asymptomatic.

38. **The answer is L.** *Pneumocystis carinii* is the most common cause of pneumonia in immunosuppressed patients with AIDS.

39. **The answer is F.** *Entamoeba histolytica* is the most important parasite that causes colonic ulceration.

40. **The answer is F.** So-called amebic abscess of the liver, although it does not contain pus, is an important complication of *amebiasis*.

41. **The answer is J.** *Naegleria fowleri* is a free-living ameba in the soil that causes rhinitis. By invading the olfactory nerves, it reaches the meninges and the brain.

42. **The answer is E.** *Cryptosporidiosis*, an enteric infection in animals, has been recognized in patients with AIDS.

43. **The answer is G.** *Giardia lamblia* is a harmless commensal that causes no symptoms in most persons. However, in some people, especially in children, *Giardia* causes diarrhea and nonspecific gastrointestinal symptoms. The organisms can be recovered from stool specimens, duodenal aspirates, or intestinal biopsies.

44. **The answer is B.** *Aspergillus* infection can produce fungus balls in dilated bronchi, composed of hyphae of the fungus intermixed with mucus and cell debris.

45. **The answer is B.** *Aspergillus* tends to invade blood vessels and cause thrombosis, with resulting angiocentric infarction. Necrotic tissue is more easily invaded than normal tissue.

46. **The answer is C.** Oral thrush is typically a mucosal *candidiasis* and is particularly common in malnourished children or those raised under unhygienic conditions.

47. **The answer is N.** Ulcerated nodules on the skin, with satellite nodules along the lymphatics, are typically caused by *Sporothrix schenkii*, a ubiquitous fungus in the soil that enters the skin with thorns or splinters.

48. **The answer is H.** *Histoplasmosis* causes pulmonary granulomatous lesions that calcify and are radiologically indistinguishable from tuberculosis.

49. **The answer is R.** *Trychophyton* infects the skin and hair, causing superficial skin mycoses.

50. **The answer is Q.** *Trichinella spiralis* larvae invade the muscle, where they cause myositis and destruction of muscle fibers. The most commonly involved muscles are those of the extremities and diaphragm.

51. **The answer is O.** In patients with compromised immunity, the infective larvae of *Strongyloides stercoralis* penetrate through the intestinal mucosa and cause hyperinfection, marked by widespread dissemination of the parasites throughout the body.

52. **The answer is A.** *Ascariasis*, the most common helminthic infestation, is often asymptomatic. However, worms in the intestine may cause various symptoms and even obstruct the intestine.

53. **The answer is M.** Schistosomiasis in humans involves three species: *S. haematobium*, which infects the urinary bladder, and *S. mansoni* and *S. japonicum*, which cause liver disease. The eggs of *S. haematobium* are most prominent in the urinary bladder, urethra, and seminal vesicles, but they may also be found in the colon or even in the lungs. The incidence of carcinoma of the urinary bladder is increased in persons who harbor *S. haematobium*.

54. **The answer is D.** Biliary infestation is a feature of *Clonorchis sinensis (Opistorchis sinensis)* infection. The duodenal cercariae enter through the papilla of Vater, migrate upward into the liver, and mature into adult flukes in the distal bile ducts.

55. **The answer is D.** The incidence of cholangiocarcinoma is increased in Chinese infected with *C. sinensis*.

Chapter 10

Blood Vessels

Questions

DIRECTIONS: Match each numbered statement with the most appropriate lettered item. Each lettered item can be used once, more than once, or not at all.

Vascular Diseases

A. Arteriolosclerosis, hyaline
B. Arteriolosclerosis, hyperplastic with fibrinoid necrosis
C. Atherosclerosis
D. Behçet disease
E. Buerger disease
F. Churg-Strauss disease
G. Fibromuscular dysplasia of arteries
H. Giant cell granulomatous arteritis
I. Henoch-Schönlein purpura
J. Hypersensitivity vasculitis
K. Kawasaki disease
L. Mönckeberg medial sclerosis
M. Polyarteritis nodosa
N. Raynaud phenomenon
O. Syphilis
P. Systemic microembolism
Q. Typhus
R. Wegener granulomatosis

_____ 1. A 30-year-old woman periodically took sulfa drugs for recurrent cystitis. Five days following the beginning of the most recent therapy, she developed a widespread skin rash. Leukocytoclastic vasculitis involving dermal venules was diagnosed by skin biopsy.

_____ 2. A 45-year-old man complained of nasal bleeding and progressive cough. He suffered from necrotizing vasculitis of the nose and lung and renal failure. A test for c-ANCA was positive.

_____ 3. A 3-year-old child presented with high fever, rash, conjunctival and oral lesions, and lymphadenitis. The child was hospitalized because of the sudden onset heart failure, which was unresponsive to treatment. The child died and the autopsy disclosed a coronary artery aneurysm.

_____ 4. A 30-year-old man known to be a heavy smoker developed gangrene of the leg, which had to be amputated. Intraluminal thrombi associated with microabscesses in the wall of medium-sized arteries were found in the resected leg. The inflammation extended from arteries to neighboring veins and nerves.

_____ 5. A 60-year-old man underwent amputation of an arm for a muscle tumor. The pathologist found calcification in the wall of the radial artery, which otherwise appeared unremarkable.

_____ 6. Subungual and conjunctival hemorrhages occurred in a patient with bacterial endocarditis.

_____ 7. A skin rash, blood in the stool, and hematuria developed in a 6-year-old child. A skin biopsy showed deposits of IgA in the walls of small blood vessels.

_____ 8. Systemic vasculitis, involving medium-sized arteries of the kidney, and accompanied by eosinophilia was diagnosed in a 19-year-old man with asthma.

_____ 9. An 80-year-old man complained of headaches; a biopsy showed temporal arteritis.

_____ 10. Blanching of the fingers upon exposure to cold was noticed in a 30-year-old, otherwise healthy woman.

_____ 11. A 40-year-old man presented with muscle pain, tingling of fingers, and bilateral arm weakness. A muscle biopsy revealed vasculitis with fibrinoid necrosis affecting small and medium-sized muscular arteries.

_____ 12. Unilateral stenosis of renal artery was found to be the cause of hypertension in a 17-year-old man. In the wall of the narrowed renal artery, smooth muscle cells were replaced by fibroblasts and myofibroblasts.

_____ 13. A 50-year-old man complained of fever, malaise, abdominal pain, bloody urine, and loss of sensation in both legs. Serologic findings were inconclusive, but a positive p-ANCA test suggested a possible autoimmune disease. Angiography revealed microaneurysms of the renal and intrarenal arteries. A sural nerve biopsy disclosed vasculitis involving muscular arteries.

_____ 14. A purpuric rash developed overnight without any obvious causes in a 30-year-old woman with Sjögren syndrome.

_____ 15. A 25-year-old man presented with dyspnea and hemoptysis. Cavitary lesions were found in both lungs by x-ray. An infectious disease work-up gave negative results. Tests for antinuclear antigens (_ANA_) and antineutrophilic cytoplasmic antibodies in a cytoplasmic pattern (c-ANCA) were positive. The p-ANCA test was negative. The patient responded well to immunosuppressive therapy with cyclophosphamide.

_____ 16. A 20-year-old woman complained of double vision, fainting spells, tingling of the fingers of the left hand, and numbness of the fingers of the right hand. The blood pressures measured in the left and right arms were 150/100 and 110/90 mm Hg, respectively. She developed pneumonia and died. At autopsy the aorta had a thickened wall and showed fragmentation of elastic fibers and vasculitis.

_____ 17. Oral aphthous ulcers, conjunctivitis, and shallow ulcerations of the mucosa of the glans penis were found in a 40-year-old man.

_____ 18. A fusiform aneurysm of the abdominal aorta in a 70-year-old man was surgically resected and replaced by a graft.

_____ 19. An aneurysm of the thoracic aorta was found at autopsy of a 60-year-old man. The vasa vasorum of the aorta were surrounded by lymphocytes and plasma cells, and the intima of the aorta showed fine scarring, imparting a tree-bark appearance.

_____ 20. A 40-year-old man had a purpuric skin rash, generalized pneumonia and elevated liver function tests. He died and intracellular pathogens up to 1 μm in length were found in endothelial cells.

_____ 21. A 50-year-old diabetic woman had a kidney biopsy. The renal arterioles had thickened eosinophilic walls.

_____ 22. A 30-year-old African-American man died of brain hemorrhage complicating a bout of hypertension of sudden onset. Renal arterioles were markedly narrowed due to proliferation of smooth muscle cells in an onion-ring pattern with focal fibrin deposition.

A n s w e r s

1. **The answer is J.** *Hypersensitivity vasculitis,* which is often drug-induced, typically presents in form of a skin rash or purpura. Skin lesions are related to a necrotizing immune-mediated inflammation of dermal venules. The leukocytic infiltrates and fibrinoid necrosis of vessels lead to rupture of the vessel walls and pinpoint, perivascular, dermal hemorrhages. Because the white blood cells in the vessels tend to die and fragment, this vasculitis is called leukocytoclastic (Greek, *klastos* means "broken" or "fragmented").

2. **The answer is R.** Necrotizing granulomatous vasculitis involving the upper and lower respiratory tract and the kidneys is a triad typically encountered in *Wegener granulomatosis*. This autoimmune disease of unknown etiology is typically accompanied by the appearance of cytoplasmic antineutrophil cytoplasm antibodies (c-ANCA).

3. **The answer is K.** *Kawasaki disease,* or mucocutaneous lymph node syndrome, is a vasculitis of unknown etiology that presents with fever, skin rash, mucosal inflammation and lymph node enlargement. The disease usually has a self-limited course but may involve the coronary arteries and lead to aneurysm formation. Death caused by heart failure occurs in 1% to 2% of cases.

4. **The answer is E.** Occlusive vasculopathy of young and middle-aged men who smoke is a feature of *Buerger disease,* or thromboangitis obliterans. The lesions typically occur in medium-sized arteries of the extremities, which also show signs of inflammation and intramural abscess formation. Inflammation may extend to adjacent veins and nerves.

5. **The answer is L.** Calcification of the media of large and medium-sized arteries of older persons not otherwise affected by atherosclerosis is typical of *Mönckeberg medial sclerosis*. These arterial changes are usually asymptomatic.

6. **The answer is P.** Solitary skin or mucosal hemorrhages in patients with bacterial endocarditis represent hemorrhagic infarcts caused by small *emboli*. A widespread skin rash is, however, a sign of vasculitis, mediated by immune complexes that form in response to valvular infection.

7. **The answer is I.** Purpura associated with gastrointestinal bleeding and glomerulonephritis in a child suggests the diagnosis of *Henoch-Schönlein purpura*, an immune-mediated vasculitis. Deposits of IgA in small blood vessels are diagnostic of the disorder.

8. **The answer is F.** Systemic vasculitis, eosinophilia, and asthma are typical of *Churg-Strauss syndrome*, also known as *allergic granulomatosis* and *angiitis*. The vasculitis is similar to the lesions of polyarteritis nodosa or Wegener granulomatosis. Patients suffering from these two diseases, however, do not have asthma or eosinophilia.

9. **The answer is H.** Temporal arteritis presents histologically as a *giant cell granulomatous* inflammation, which destroys the media of the temporal artery and predisposes to thrombosis. Headaches, typically in form of throbbing temporal pain, and visual problems may appear. Often a palpable tortuous and swollen temporal artery may be the only physical finding.

10. **The answer is N.** Blanching of fingers upon exposure to cold suggests the diagnosis of *Raynaud phenomenon*. This condition occurs in a variety of vascular and autoimmune diseases (e.g., SLE or scleroderma).

11. **The answer is M.** Inflammation with fibrinoid necrosis of muscular arteries is typical of *polyarteritis nodosa*.

12. **The answer is G.** Narrowing of the lumen by proliferating fibroblasts and myofibroblasts is a typical feature of *fibromuscular dysplasia* of a renal artery. Renal ischemia leads to increased secretion of renin and hypertension.

13. **The answer is M.** Vasculitis involving muscular arteries and resulting in microaneurysms is a feature of *polyarteritis nodosa.* Many patients have p-ANCA, but this serologic test is not diagnostic. The diagnosis is usually made by biopsy of the skin, muscle, peripheral nerves, or the most affected internal organs (the kidney in this case).

14. **The answer is J.** Purpura or a skin rash in a patient with a known autoimmune disease, such as Sjögren syndrome or SLE, can usually be related to *hypersensitivity vasculitis*, which is caused by the deposition of immune complexes in dermal venules.

15. **The answer is R.** The clinical and laboratory data, together with a good response to therapy, suggest that this patient had *Wegener granulomatosis* in a "limited form" (i.e., involving only the lungs). c-ANCA antibodies, recognizing proteinase 3 of azurophilic granules in neutrophils, are typical of Wegener granulomatosis but are also found in polyarteritis nodosa. The p-ANCA test recognizes antibodies to myeloperoxidase and is more common in vasculitis limited to the kidneys.

16. **The answer is H.** Ischemic cerebral episodes in a young woman and a differential between the blood pressure in the left and right arm suggest Takayasu disease, a *granulomatous giant cell* arteritis involving the aorta and its major branches. More than 90% of patients are women under 30 years of age. Narrowing of the arteries accounts for ischemic episodes and the "pulseless disease."

17. **The answer is D.** Oral and genital ulcers associated with conjunctivitis and signs of systemic disease are features of *Behçet disease*. The cause of this necrotizing inflammation of small blood vessels is not known.

18. **The answer is C.** *Atherosclerosis* is the most common cause of aortic aneurysms in general. In the elderly, almost all of the aneurysms of the abdominal aorta are related to atherosclerosis.

19. **The answer is O.** Teritary *syphilis* typically involves the vasa vasorum of the aorta. Destructive lesions of the aortic wall are related to obliterative vasculitis of the vasa vasorum and predispose to aneurysm formation, typically of the aortic arch.

20. **The answer is Q.** *Rickettsia prowazekii* is the causative agent of *typhus fever*. Like all other Rickettsiae, it invades the endothelial cells, causing vasculitis and hemorrhages from ruptured small blood vessels.

21. **The answer is A.** Diabetes leads to *hyaline arteriolosclerosis,* which is prominent in the kidneys.

22. **The answer is B.** Malignant hypertension is associated with *hyperplastic arteriolosclerosis,* which may also show focal fibrinoid necrosis.

Chapter 11

The Heart

Questions

DIRECTIONS: Match each numbered statement with the most appropriate lettered item. Each lettered item can be used once, more than once, or not at all.

Congenital Heart Disease

A. Aortic stenosis
B. Atrial septal defect, ostium primum type
C. Atrial septal defect, ostium secundum type
D. Atrioventricular septal defect
E. Coarctation of aorta, postductal (juxtaductal)
F. Coarctation of aorta, preductal
G. Patent ductus arteriosus
H. Pulmonary stenosis
I. Tetralogy of Fallot
J. Transposition of great vessels
K. Truncus arteriosus communis
L. Ventricular septal defect

_____ 1. Isolated defect in the middle portion of the atrial septum involving the limbus of the foramen ovale. It accounts for 90% of all atrial septal defects.

_____ 2. The most common congenital heart defect, when large enough, leads to biventricular cardiac hypertrophy but not to cyanosis.

_____ 3. Persistent embryonic structure connecting the pulmonary artery with the aorta. It is kept open by prostaglandins (PGE_2) and can be closed medically by inhibitors of prostaglandin synthesis, such as indomethacin.

_____ 4. The aorta and pulmonary artery are not separated from each other and form a single vessel overriding a ventricular septal defect. This vessel receives blood from both ventricles.

_____ 5. The most common cyanotic congenital heart defect. It comprises pulmonary stenosis, ventricular septal defect, dextroposition of the aorta, and right ventricular hypertrophy.

_____ **6.** The aorta arises from the right ventricle and the pulmonary artery from the left ventricle, resulting in early cyanosis. The anomaly formerly had a 90% mortality rate within the first year of life, but with modern surgery 90% of affected children survive.

_____ **7.** Isolated narrowing of the aorta caused by a ridgelike fold in the wall of the aorta opposite to the ligamentum arteriosum. It is associated with hypertension in the upper extremities and low pressure in both legs.

DIRECTIONS: Match each numbered statement with the most appropriate lettered item. Each lettered item can be used once, more than once, or not at all.

Heart Diseases

A. Calcific aortic stenosis
B. Carcinoid heart disease
C. Cardiomyopathy, dilated
D. Cardiomyopathy, hypertrophic
E. Cardiomyopathy, restrictive
F. Endocarditis, acute, infective
G. Endocarditis, chronic
H. Endocarditis, nonbacterial, thrombotic
I. Mitral valve prolapse
J. Myocardial infarction, subendocardial
K. Myocardial infarction, transmural
L. Myocarditis
M. Myxoma
N. Pericarditis
O. Rhabdomyoma
P. Rheumatic heart disease
Q. Ventricular aneurysm

_____ **8.** A 40-year-old woman developed a flulike syndrome, with prominent muscle pains. Owing to palpitations and a "strange feeling around my heart," she consulted her physician, who noticed tachycardia and irregular beats. The patient died of uncontrollable arrhythmias. At autopsy foci of myocardial cell necrosis were surrounded by lymphocytes and macrophages.

_____ **9.** A 45-year-old Vietnamese immigrant who had active pulmonary tuberculosis developed shortness of breath, swelling of the legs, and enlargement of the liver. Auscultation revealed friction rub. The cardiac silhouette was enlarged, and the usual markings of the heart were not visible radiologically.

_____ **10.** A 60-year-old man suffered a myocardial infarction, and a left ventricular "bulge" was noticed on x-ray 6 months later. The "bulge" did not contract during systole.

_____ **11.** During surgery for mitral valve stenosis in a 35-year-old Haitian man, the surgeon obtained a biopsy of the left atrial appendage. The myocardium contained aggregates of macrophages arranged around centrally located deposits of fibrin (Aschoff bodies).

_____ **12.** A 60-year-old man with a remarkably enlarged heart had signs of heart failure and an increased end-diastolic pressure. Endomyocardial biopsy of the right ventricle revealed eosinophilic deposits between the cardiac myocytes.

_____ **13.** A 20-year-old woman with a history of intravenous drug abuse presented with chills, fever, and malaise. A systolic murmur was heard over the aortic valve. Before treatment could be instituted, she suffered a stroke and died 2 days later. A brain abscess was found at autopsy.

_____ **14.** A 40-year-old man with congenital hyperlipidemia underwent resection of an aortic aneurysm, after which he developed cardiac failure. EKG showed "non-Q-wave" infarct. Despite all treatment, he died 2 days later. An autopsy disclosed marked narrowing of the coronary arteries but no occlusion. Foci of myocardial necrosis were found circumferentially around the lumina of both ventricles.

_____ **15.** A 30-year-old woman with systemic lupus erythematosus developed a murmur over the mitral valve, after which she had a stroke. She had no fever, and blood cultures were negative.

_____ **16.** A 5-cm mass that obstructed the mitral orifice in a "ball/valve" fashion was removed surgically from the left atrium of a 40-year-old man. Histologically, it was composed of elongated and stellate cells, embedded in a loose, edematous stroma.

_____ **17.** A 78-year-old man with left ventricular hypertrophy had cardiac surgery, and a hard, markedly deformed aortic valve was resected. An artificial valve was installed in its place.

_____ **18.** Cardiologic examination revealed pulmonic stenosis and tricuspid regurgitation in a 45-year-old woman. She had an enlarged liver, and blood tests showed increased urinary 5-hydroxyindolacetic acid and elevated chromogranin-A.

_____ **19.** A 60-year-old man was hospitalized for thrombosis of the left main coronary artery. He died 5 days later of cardiac tamponade.

_____ **20.** A 50-year-old man underwent heart transplantation for low-output cardiac failure that was unresponsive to medical treatment. The heart weighed 600 g (normal up to 350 g) and showed no coronary atherosclerosis. Histologically, the myocardium showed signs of hypertrophy and foci of myocardial fibrosis but no inflammation.

DIRECTIONS: Choose the one best answer.

_____ **21.** Myocardial infarct involving the posterior portion of the interventricular septum is caused by an occlusion of which coronary artery?

A. Right
B. Left anterior descending
C. Left circumflex
D. Left diagonal
E. Obtuse

_____ 22. Circumferential subendocardial infarcts are typically a consequence of

A. coronary spasm.
B. inadequate anastomotic circulation.
C. hypoperfusion of the heart in shock.
D. cardiac tamponade.
E. mitral stenosis.

_____ 23. What is the most common cause of death during the first 2 hours after an acute myocardial infarction?

A. Arrhythmia
B. Loss of myosin from injured cells
C. Loss of troponin T from necrotic cells
D. Loss of calcium from sarcoplasmic reticulum
E. Rupture of the myocardium

_____ 24. What is the most likely age of a myocardial infarct that is infiltrated with neutrophils?

A. Less than 6 hours
B. Three days
C. Seven days
D. Fourteen days
E. Six weeks

_____ 25. Which of the following enzymes is increased first in the blood after acute myocardial infarction?

A. Alkaline phosphatase
B. Acid phosphatase
C. Alanine aminotransferase
D. Aspartate aminotransferase
E. Creatine kinase

_____ 26. Which of the following is the most likely cardiac consequence of hyperthyroidism?

A. Subendocardial necrosis
B. Coronary spasm
C. Anteroseptal infarct
D. Tachycardia
E. Marantic endocarditis

_____ 27. The Jones major criteria for diagnosing rheumatic fever include all the following *except*

A. carditis.
B. aortitis.
C. polyarthritis.
D. chorea.
E. erythema marginatum.

_____ 28. Which of the following diseases is most often associated with nonbacterial thrombotic endocarditis?

A. Rubella
B. Syphilis
C. Carcinoma of the stomach
D. Intestinal carcinoid metastatic to the liver
E. Kawasaki disease

_____ **29.** Myocarditis is a common complication of infection with

A. *Schistosoma mansoni.*
B. *Treponema pallidum.*
C. *Trichuris trichiura.*
D. *Trypanosoma cruzi.*
E. *Pneumocystis carinii.*

_____ **30.** Asymmetrical septal hypertrophy is found in

A. alcoholic cardiomyopathy.
B. amyloidosis of the heart.
C. ischemic cardiomyopathy.
D. congenital hypertrophic cardiomyopathy.
E. dilated cardiomyopathy.

Answers

1. **The answer is C.** *Atrial septal defect* (ASD), ostium secundum type, is located in the middle portion of the atrial septum, in contrast to an ostium primum defect, which is positioned in the lower part. A sinus venosus defect of the septum is positioned in the upper part of the septum. ASD ostium secundum type represents a true defect of the valve or limbus of the fetal fossa ovalis and should be distinguished from patent foramen ovale, which is found in 30% of normal persons. This anomaly accounts for 90% of all ASD. In most instances it occurs as an isolated defect, but it may be associated with other cardiac defects.

2. **The answer is L.** *Ventricular septal defect* involving the membranous portion of the interventricular septum is the most common congenital heart defect, accounting for 30% of all cases. It occurs most often as an isolated defect, but it may be also associated with other cardiac anomalies. It is a regular feature of tetralogy of Fallot.

3. **The answer is G.** *Patent ductus arteriosus* (PDA) represents an incomplete closure of the fetal blood vessel that shunts the blood from the pulmonary artery to the aorta, thereby bypassing the fetal lungs. Ductus arteriosus is kept open by PGE_2, and injection of indomethacin can lead to its closure. A large PDA must be closed surgically or by catheterization techniques.

4. **The answer is K.** *Truncus arteriosus communis* results from incomplete partitioning of the main fetal blood vessel (truncus arteriosus). During normal development this vessel is divided by the spiral septum into the pulmonary artery and aorta. Abnormal hemodynamics cause early death owing to heart failure. Increased pulmonary blood flow is also associated with recurrent respiratory infections. A few persons who survive longer develop pulmonary hypertension.

5. **The answer is I.** *Tetralogy of Fallot* (*tetra* means "four" in Greek) is defined by four anatomic changes (pulmonary stenosis, ventricular septal defect, dextroposition of the aorta, and right ventricular hypertrophy). It accounts for 10% of all congenital heart defects and is the most common cyanotic congenital heart disease. Cyanosis, which appears shortly after birth or early in infancy, develops because of the right-to-left shunting of venous blood from the right ventricle into the dextra-

posed aorta. The latter overrides the septal defect and receives blood from both ventricles. Narrowing of the pulmonary artery impedes the entry of blood into the lung, thereby increasing the pressure in the right ventricle.

6. **The answer is J.** *Transposition of great vessels* results from abnormal partitioning of the fetal truncus arteriosus communis by the spiral septum. This partitioning is associated with a rotation during which the ostium of the pulmonary artery assumes an anterior position on the right side and the orifice of the aorta takes a posterior position on the left.

   Abnormal morphogenesis during fetal life that results in abnormal positioning of the pulmonary artery and the aorta causes early cyanosis because the aorta receives venous blood from the right ventricle. This anomaly was associated with early death in 90% of infants, but modern surgery has remarkably improved survival, and 90% of affected children can be saved.

7. **The answer is E.** *Coarctation of the aorta* of the postductal type occurs in an isolated form or with other cardiac anomalies that limit cardiac output (e.g., bicuspid aortic valve). In contrast to preductal coarctation, which becomes symptomatic early in life (hence called *infantile coarctation*), the postductal (also known as *juxtaductal*) variant may be asymptomatic or associated only with symptoms of late onset. Narrowing of the lumen limits blood flow to those parts of the body below the aortic arch. As a result, anastomoses develop between the major arteries originating above the coarctation and those below it. Blood pressure measured in the arms is high, whereas that in the lower extremities is low.

8. **The answer is L.** *Myocarditis* (i.e., inflammation of the myocardium) is associated with necrosis of cardiac myocytes and is often caused by viruses. Coxsackievirus is one of the more common pathogens.

9. **The answer is N.** *Pericarditis* is the most common cardiac manifestation of tuberculosis. It is rare in Western countries but is still prevalent in underdeveloped countries of Africa and Asia.

10. **The answer is Q.** *Ventricular aneurysm* is a localized dilatation of the left ventricle, which occurs at the site of a healed, transmural, myocardial infarct. Intraventricular blood exerts pressure on the scar tissue that replaces the necrotic myocardium, thereby causing it to bulge outward. Such aneurysms often contain mural thrombi.

11. **The answer is P.** Aschoff bodies are diagnostic of *rheumatic heart disease*, a pancarditis that may affect any part of the heart. Stenosis or insufficiency of the aortic and mitral valves is the most significant chronic complication.

12. **The answer is E.** Amyloidosis causes *restrictive cardiomyopathy*, characterized by reduced diastolic filling. Other causes of restrictive cardiomyopathy are hemochromatosis, sarcoidosis, endomyocardial fibroelastosis, and myocardial fibrosis.

13. **The answer is F.** Signs of septicemia and cardiac murmurs in a person addicted to intravenous drug abuse are indicative of *bacterial (infective) endocarditis*. Infected vegetations may detach from the valves and embolize through the arterial circulation to various organs, such as the brain or kidneys, where they cause infarcts. Bacteria in the embolus invade the infarct, transforming it into an abscess.

14. **The answer is J.** *Subendocardial infarcts* typically present as foci of myocyte necrosis around the cardiac chambers. Such infarcts are caused by hypoperfusion of the myocardium and are not limited to particular anatomic sites supplied by specific coronary arteries.

15. **The answer is H.** Libman-Sacks endocarditis, a complication of SLE, is a *nonbacterial endocarditis* most often involving the undersurface of mitral valve. The verrucous vegetations consist of fibrin. Although some vegetations may contain diagnostic hematoxylin bodies, they are usually indistinguishable from other nonbacterial vegetations, as in marantic or rheumatic endocarditis.

16. **The answer is M.** *Myxoma*, the most common primary cardiac tumor, presents as a pedunculated, intraatrial mass, usually attached to the mitral valve. It is a benign tumor composed of fibroblast-like cells that are surrounded by a loose, edematous ("myxomatous") stroma.

17. **The answer is A.** *Calcific aortic stenosis* is a degenerative disease of old age, which is the most common cause of aortic valvular stenosis. The cause of valvular calcification is obscure.

18. **The answer is B.** *Carcinoid heart disease* typically affects the right heart, causing changes in the pulmonary and tricuspid valves. It is associated with intestinal carcinoids that have metastasized to the liver. In that location they discharge serotonin and other biologically active polypeptides directly into the venous blood. Intestinal carcinoids that have not metastasized to the liver do not cause carcinoid heart disease, because their secretions are released into the portal venous system, after which they are degraded by the liver and do not reach the heart. The left heart is not affected in carcinoid syndrome because the lung is rich in monoamine oxidase and has the capacity to remove bioactive amines.

19. **The answer is K.** Hemopericardium is a lethal complication of *transmural myocardial infarction*. Rupture of the left ventricle usually occurs during the first week after coronary occlusion, when the infarcted myocardium is particularly soft.

20. **The answer is C.** *Dilated cardiomyopathy* is a term that describes a markedly enlarged and dilated heart that shows no evidence of coronary heart disease or valvular disease. This end-stage heart disease could result from previous viral myocarditis or toxic injury, but in most cases the cause remains unknown.

21. **The answer is A.** Posterior septal infarcts of the posterior wall and posterior septum are caused by occlusion of the *right coronary artery*.

22. **The answer is C.** Circumferential subendocardial infarcts are caused by *hypoperfusion* of the myocardium, as occurs in shock, near drowning, and asphyxia, for example.

23. **The answer is A.** *Arrhythmia* is the most common cause of early death after myocardial infarction.

24. **The answer is B.** Neutrophils appear in the infarcted myocardium approximately 24 hours after coronary artery occlusion and are most prominent *after 2–4 days.* Thereafter, neutrophils are replaced by macrophages and granulation tissue.

25. **The answer is E.** An increased level of *creatine kinase* in the blood is an early biochemical sign of myocardial infarction.

26. **The answer is D.** Hyperthyroidism causes *tachycardia.*

27. **The answer is B.** The Jones major criteria of rheumatic fever include carditis, polyarthritis, chorea, erythema marginatum, and subcutaneous nodules. *Aortitis is not a feature of rheumatic fever.*

28. **The answer is C.** Nonbacterial thrombotic endocarditis, also known as marantic endocarditis, is typically found in emaciated *persons with cancer.*

29. **The answer is D.** *Trypanosoma cruzi,* the protozoon that causes Chagas disease, tends to invade cardiac myocytes and to cause myocarditis.

30. **The answer is D.** Asymmetrical septal hypertrophy is a typical feature of *congenital hypertrophic cardiomyopathy,* which is inherited as an autosomal dominant trait.

Chapter 12

Lung Diseases

Questions

DIRECTIONS: Match each numbered statement with the most appropriate lettered item. Each lettered item can be used once, more than once, or not at all.

Lung Diseases

    A. Abscess of the lung
    B. Adult respiratory distress syndrome
    C. Asbestosis
    D. Asthma
    E. Atelectasis
    F. Bronchiectasis
    G. Bronchitis, acute
    H. Bronchopneumonia
    I. Coal workers' pneumoconiosis
    J. Emphysema
    K. Goodpasture syndrome
    L. Hypersensitivity pneumonitis
    M. Pneumonia, atypical
    N. Pneumonia, lobar
    O. Sarcoidosis
    P. Silicosis
    Q. Tuberculosis
    R. Usual interstitial pneumonia
    S. Wegener granulomatosis

_____ **1.** A 63-year-old man was diagnosed with small cell carcinoma of the left main bronchus, for which he received chemotherapy. During the treatment period he became febrile and developed leukocytosis. His cough worsened and he began expectorating large amounts of mucopurulent sputum. X-ray disclosed a localized lucent area with a distinct air/fluid level, surrounded by a density distal to the tumor mass.

_____ **2.** A 20-year-old woman with cystic fibrosis died of recurrent pneumonia. The bronchi of lungs were dilated and contained prominent mucoropurulent plugs. These cylindrical bronchial lesions are known as ...

_____ 3. A 60-year-old stone mason complained of shortness of breath, which had become worse during the last year. Multiple small nodular shadows were seen in both of his lungs, and functional studies revealed reduced pulmonary compliance and diffusing capacity. He died of heart failure. An autopsy revealed numerous small fibrotic nodules, which contained birefingent crystals.

_____ 4. A 35-year-old black woman had fever and joint pains for 3 months. A chest x-ray revealed symmetrical enlargement of the hilar lymph nodes. A transbronchial biopsy revealed noncaseating granulomas. Blood levels of serum angiotensin converting enzyme (ACE) were elevated.

_____ 5. A 60-year-old man was salvaged from a burning house. About 70% of his body surface was burned, and he died of pulmonary insufficiency after 3 days. Histologically, the alveoli contained proteinaceous material and hyaline membranes.

_____ 6. A 20-year-old man complained of low-grade fever and cough for a month. The sputum contained acid-fast bacilli, and an x-ray revealed findings "consistent with a Ghon complex."

_____ 7. A 40-year-old chronic alcoholic was hospitalized in severe respiratory distress. He coughed constantly and expectorated reddish-yellow sputum. X-rays revealed bilateral, diffuse, pulmonary consolidation. He died from streptococcal sepsis. At autopsy both lungs were airless, heavy, and consolidated. Histologically, almost all alveoli were filled with neutrophils and fibrin.

_____ 8. A 50-year-old pigeon fancier complained of bouts of fever, shortness of breath, cough, and chest tightness. Blood tests revealed antibodies to bird proteins. A lung biopsy demonstrated poorly formed granulomas composed of epithelioid macrophages and multinucleated giant cells.

_____ 9. A 75-year-old man who worked in a shipyard died of chronic lung disease. Pulmonary fibrosis and pleural plaques were found at autopsy. Numerous brown beaded bodies were found in the pulmonary parenchyma.

_____ 10. A 40-year-old man with α_1-antitrypsin deficiency died of complications of cirrhosis. At autopsy his lungs showed widespread loss of alveolar septa, imparting a "cotton candy–like" appearance.

DIRECTIONS: Match each numbered statement with the most appropriate lettered item. Each lettered item can be used once, more than once, or not at all.

Lung Tumors

A. Adenocarcinoma
B. Bronchioloalveolar carcinoma
C. Carcinoid
D. Eosinophilic granuloma of the lung
E. Large cell undifferentiated carcinoma

F. Mesothelioma
G. Metastatic carcinoma
H. Small cell carcinoma
I. Squamous cell carcinoma

_____ 11. A hilar tumor composed of keratinizing cells connected by inter-cellular bridges and desmosomes.

_____ 12. A subpleural mass in the upper lobe, caused puckering of the overlying pleura, was composed of cuboidal cells, forming irregular, glandlike, structures in a densely collagenous stroma.

_____ 13. A bulky mass within the pulmonary parenchyma was composed of large cells, arranged without any distinct pattern, scattered giant cells, and broad areas of necrosis and hemorrhage.

_____ 14. A tumor diffusely infiltrated the lung parenchyma and was composed of well-differentiated, mucus-producing, columnar neoplastic cells lining alveolar spaces. No tumors were found in other organs.

_____ 15. A malignant hilar tumor was composed of cells with round or oval hyperchomatic nuclei and scant cytoplasm. Broad areas of necrosis were present. Electron microscopy disclosed neuroendocrine granules in the cytoplasm of some tumor cells.

_____ 16. A polypoid nodule protruding into a lobar bronchus was composed of ribbons and nests of small cells, with uniform round nuclei filled with finely dispersed chromatin. Electron microscopy revealed that the tumor cells contained numerous neuroendocrine granules.

_____ 17. A biphasic pleural tumor was composed of cuboidal epithelial cells that lined glandlike and tubulelike structures and spindle-shaped cells similar to those of a fibrosarcoma.

_____ 18. Multiple, bilateral round, "cannon ball" masses were found radiologically in both lungs of an elderly man. Histologically, the nodules were composed of glandlike structures.

_____ 19. An infiltrating mass with cystic spaces was resected from the upper lobe of a young man. Histologically, it was composed of Langerhans cells and scattered eosinophils.

DIRECTIONS: Choose the one best answer.

_____ 20. Acute upper respiratory tract obstruction, known as croup, is most often caused by
A. viruses.
B. bacteria.
C. fungi.
D. protozoa.
E. mycoplasma.

_____ 21. The most common consequence of pneumothorax is
A. emphysema.
B. atelectasis.
C. empyema.
D. pyothorax.
E. diffuse alveolar damage.

_____ **22.** A syndrome marked by minor respiratory symptoms of insidious onset and accompanied by radiographic evidence of interstitial infiltration and a mild intraalveolar exudation is typically caused by
   A. *Streptococcus pneumoniae.*
   ʾB. *Mycoplasma pneumoniae.*
   C. *Klebsiella pneumoniae.*
   D. *Staphylococcus aureus.*
   E. *Mycobacterium tuberculosis.*

_____ **23.** Multiple thrombi in small branches of the pulmonary artery are typical of infection with
   A. adenovirus.
   B. parainfluenza virus.
   C. mucormycosis.
   D. *Pneumocystis carinii.*
   E. *Hemophilus influenzae.*

_____ **24.** Asthma in children who have a positive skin test to a suspected antigen is mediated by
   A. IgE.
   B. IgA.
   C. IgG.
   D. IgM.
   E. IgD.

_____ **25.** The most important cause of emphysema in the United States is
   A. air pollution.
   B. cigarette smoking.
   C. α_1-antitrypsin deficiency.
   D. cystic fibrosis.
   E. human immunodeficiency virus.

_____ **26.** The primary defense to tuberculosis is mediated by
   A. IgA.
   B. IgE.
   C. IgG and IgM.
   D. T cells.
   E. NK cells.

_____ **27.** A lung biopsy in a 50-year-old man with a chronic lung disease of unknown etiology revealed some alveoli were normal, whereas others were fibrotic and infiltrated sparsely with lymphocytes. These findings are most consistent with the diagnosis of
   A. usual interstitial pneumonia.
   B. desquamative interstitial pneumonia.
   C. Wegener granulomatosis.
   D. Churg-Strauss syndrome.
   E. Goodpasture syndrome.

_____ **28.** All the following diseases are examples of extrinsic allergic alveolitis *except*

    A. silicosis.
    B. bagassosis.
    C. turkey handler's disease.
    D. farmer's lung.
    E. maple bark stripper's disease.

_____ **29.** Therapeutic aspiration of a massive pleural effusion under sterile circumstances may cause

    A. atelectasis.
    B. emphysema.
    C. bronchiectasis.
    D. pulmonary edema.
    E. emphysema.

_____ **30.** Which of the following is the most common complication of heart failure?

    A. Hydrothorax
    B. Pneumothorax
    C. Pyothorax
    D. Hemothorax
    E. Chylothorax

Answers

1. **The answer is A.** *Abscess* is a common complication of lung cancer. Infection usually occurs distal to the intrabronchial tumor mass, thereby preventing the discharge of mucus and predisposing to atelectasis. The abscess cavity is partially filled with pus and air, which accounts for the x-ray finding of an "air/fluid level." Pus from an abscess is expectorated only if the abscess is connected to a bronchus.

2. **The answer is F.** *Bronchiectasis*, or dilatation of the bronchi, is a common complication of cystic fibrosis. Bronchiectasis can be cylindrical or saccular, and the dilated bronchi are typically filled with mucopurulent material. Infection readily spreads from the bronchi into the surrounding lung parenchyma, thereby causing pneumonia.

3. **The answer is P.** *Silicosisis* is a lung disease characterized by the insidious development of fibrotic pulmonary nodules containing quartz crystals (SiO_2). It is a pneumoconiosis that develops in workers employed in quarries, stone masonry, sandblasting, and so on. The disease may be asymptomatic for prolonged periods of time or cause only mild to moderate dyspnea. Extensive pulmonary fibrosis occurs mostly in those who have also been exposed to dusts other than silica, as in coal workers' pneumoconiosis. Exposure to massive amounts of silica may cause progressive massive fibrosis.

4. **The answer is O.** *Sarcoidosis* is a disease of unknown etiology that presents with noncaseating granulomas. The hilar lymph nodes and lung are often involved. Angiotension converting enzyme (ACE) is produced by epithelioid macrophages and is elevated in the blood. Spontaneous

regression of lesions is common, but in some cases the disease causes pulmonary fibrosis and respiratory failure.

5. **The answer is B.** *Adult respiratory distress syndrome* (ARDS) is a common clinical complication of burns and is characterized by severe pulmonary edema, intra-alveolar hemorrhages, and hyaline membranes lining the damaged alveoli. The pathologic lesion is known as diffuse alveolar damage (DAD). DAD is not limited to patients with burns and may occur in other forms of shock.

6. **The answer is Q.** Primary *tuberculosis* is often asymptomatic or presents with nonspecific symptoms, such as low-grade fever, loss of appetite, and occasional spells of coughing. The Ghon complex includes parenchymal consolidation and ipsilateral enlargement of hilar lymph nodes and is often accompanied by a pleural effusion. The sputum contains *Mycobacterium tuberculosis*, which is acid-fast in smears stained by the Ziehl-Neelsen technique.

7. **The answer is N.** *Lobar pneumonia* presents with a diffuse consolidation of one or more pulmonary lobes and typically occurs in debilitated persons or those whose resistance to bacterial infection is reduced, as in alcoholics. The affected lobes appear airless and consolidated because the alveoli are filled with neutrophils.

8. **The answer is L.** *Hypersensitivity pneumonitis* may develop in response to repeated exposure to a variety of organic materials, including bird droppings, feathers, mushrooms, tree bark, and so on. Histologically, the lung contains poorly formed granulomas, which differ from the compact (solid) noncaseating granulomas of sarcoidosis and the caseating granulomas of tuberculosis or histoplasmosis.

9. **The answer is C.** *Asbestosis* is a pneumoconiosis caused by the inhalation of asbestos fibers, most often crocidolite and chrysotile. It is characterized by interstitial fibrosis, pleural effusions and plaques, and an increased incidence of mesothelioma. Asbestosis creates a high risk of lung cancer in smokers.

10. **The answer is J.** α_1-Antitrypsin deficiency is associated with the development of cirrhosis and *emphysema*. Emphysema is diffuse and is classified as panacinar.

11. **The answer is I.** *Squamous cell carcinoma* is the most common cancer of the lungs and originates from foci of squamous metaplasia in the major bronchi. The tumors are mostly located near the hilus and are composed of cells resembling those in the skin and other squamous epithelia.

12. **The answer is A.** *Adenocarcinoma* usually presents as a peripheral subpleural mass composed of neoplastic glandlike structures.

13. **The answer is E.** *Large cell undifferentiated* carcinoma is composed of atypical neoplastic cells that do not resemble any normal cells in the lung. These cells do not form glands (like adenocarcinoma) and do not undergo keratinization (like squamous carcinoma).

14. **The answer is B.** *Bronchioloalveolar carcinoma* is a primary pulmonary adenocarcinoma originating from stem cells in the terminal bronchioles. The cells may be columnar and mucus-producing or cuboidal and similar to type II pneumocytes. They tend to grow along the alveolar septa. A similar growth pattern may be seen in metastatic adenocarcinomas.

15. **The answer is H.** *Small cell carcinoma* (*also known as oat cell carcinoma*) typically forms hilar masses composed of small hyperchromatic cells that contain neuroendocrine granules.

16. **The answer is C.** *Carcinoid* tumor is a low-grade malignant tumor composed of well-differentiated neuroendocrine cells. The tumor occurs most often in the wall of a major bronchus and may protrude into its lumen.

17. **The answer is F.** *Mesothelioma* is a pleural tumor that often shows biphasic histologic features. It is composed of carcinoma-like epithelial cells and spindle-shaped cells that resemble a sarcoma.

18. **The answer is G.** *Metastatic carcinomas* typically present as multiple round masses scattered at random throughout the parenchyma of both lungs.

19. **The answer is D.** *Eosinophilic granuloma* is a mass composed of Langerhans cells and eosinophils. Localized isolated tumors have a good prognosis, but in some cases the disease may have a progressive course and cause respiratory failure.

20. **The answer is A.** Epiglottitis, or laryngotracheobronchitis, is caused by some *respiratory viruses*. It is a potentially lethal condition that presents with acute respiratory tract obstruction known as "croup."

21. **The answer is B.** Pneumothorax (i.e., the entry of air into the pleural cavity) causes collapse of the entire lung, a condition that is called *atelectasis.*

22. **The answer is B.** *Atypical pneumonia* is a term used for a syndrome marked by minor respiratory symptoms of insidious onset, which are accompanied by radiographic evidence of intra-alveolar and interstitial infiltrates. The disease produces nonspecific symptoms and fever and is characterized by a lack of leukocytosis. It is caused by *Mycoplasma pneumoniae*, viruses, or *Chlamydia.*

23. **The answer is C.** Branching fungi, including *Mucor* species, tend to invade blood vessels and cause thrombosis, with subsequent infarction of the lungs. By contrast, *Pneumocystis carinii* is noninvasive and grows inside the alveolar spaces, damaging alveolar lining cells and causing an interstitial pneumonitis. Viruses infect and damage alveolar lining cells, and bacteria cause an intra-alveolar exudate of neutrophils.

24. **The answer is A.** "Allergic asthma" is a reaginic (type I) *IgE-mediated* response of children to inhaled allergens. By contrast, "intrinsic asthma" is a disease of adults that shows a strong correlation with reactivity to allergic skin tests, which are also IgE-mediated.

25. **The answer is B.** *Cigarette smoking* is the most common cause of emphysema in the United States.

26. **The answer is D.** Individual susceptibility to tuberculosis has not been fully explained, but it does not involve antibody-mediated immune responses. The primary defense to tuberculosis is a *T-cell-mediated*, delayed hypersensitivity reaction. In tuberculosis this response produces typical granulomas, formed through the interaction of T-helper lymphocytes and macrophages.

27. **The answer is A.** *Usual interstitial pneumonia* may be caused by several unrelated pathologic processes, and the lesion evolves at different rates in different parts of the lung. Histologically, the pulmonary parenchyma shows a spectrum of changes, from almost normal alveoli to mild lymphocytic interstitial infiltration to massive obliterative alveolitis and pulmonary fibrosis.

28. **The answer is A.** All the disease listed here, except *silicosis*, represent a form of extrinsic allergic alveolitis. Acute cases of these diseases present as a hypersensitivity pneumonitis, with an exudate of polymorphonuclear leukocytes. By contrast, chronic cases of extrinsic allergic alveolitis exhibit lymphoid cells and granulomas.

29. **The answer is D.** Evacuation of the fluid from the pleural cavity relieves the pressure on the lung. Sudden expansion of the lungs may cause a rapid elevation of the pressure in the interstitial spaces, with a suction effect on the capillary fluid. Capillary fluid is drawn into the interstitial spaces and from these into the alveoli, where it appears as *pulmonary edema*.

30. **The answer is A.** The elevation of hydrostatic pressure in congestive heart failure causes transudation of fluid into the pleural cavity and, therefore, *hydrothorax*.

Chapter 13

The Gastrointestinal Tract

Questions

DIRECTIONS: **DIRECTIONS:** Match each numbered statement with the most appropriate lettered item. Each lettered item can be used once, more than once, or not at all.

Diseases of the Esophagus

A. Achalasia
B. Adenocarcinoma
C. Atresia
D. Barrett esophagus
E. Diverticulum
F. Hiatal hernia, sliding
G. Hiatal hernia, paraesophageal
H. Infectious esophagitis
I. Leiomyoma
J. Mallory-Weiss syndrome
K. Reflux esophagitis
L. Rings
M. Squamous cell carcinoma
N. Stricture
O. Varices
P. Webs

_____ 1. A 35-year-old woman complained of difficulty in swallowing, a tendency to regurgitate food, and excessive burping. No tumor inflammatory lesion, ring, or web was found during esophagogastroscopy. Manometric studies of the esophagus revealed complete absence of peristalsis, failure of the lower esophageal sphincter (LES) to relax upon swallowing, increased intra-esophageal pressure, and prominent low-amplitude, nonperistaltic contractions.

_____ 2. A 40-year-old man had esophagoscopy for dysphagia. An annular eccentric narrowing was detected in the upper third of the esophagus. Biopsy disclosed no inflammation and no neoplasia, and the lesion was considered to be composed of only esophageal mucosa.

_____   3. A 70-year-old man complained of difficulty in eating and swallowing solid food. He had lost 20 pounds over the last 6 months and felt tired and weak. Esophagogastroscopy revealed a mass in the lower third of the esophagus. Histologically, it was composed of atypical cuboidal cells lining irregular glandlike structures.

_____   4. A 40-year-old man had been treated extensively for leukemia and complained of heartburn and pain upon swallowing. A biopsy of the esophagus revealed signs of inflammation. Many nuclei of the squamous epithelium had a "ground glass appearance," and there were numerous multinucleated cells.

_____   5. A 50-year-old obese man complained of indigestion and bloating. After meals he would experience reflux of food, with a burning sensation in the chest, radiating into the throat. A hiatal hernia was diagnosed and an esophageal biopsy revealed thickening of the basal layer of the squamous epithelium, upward extension of the papillae of the lamina propria, and an increased number of lymphocytes.

DIRECTIONS: Match each numbered statement with the most appropriate lettered item. Each lettered item can be used once, more than once, or not at all.

Diseases of the Stomach

A. Acute erosive gastritis
B. Adenocarcinoma, localized
C. Chronic gastritis type A (fundal)
D. Chronic gastritis type B (antral)
E. Curling ulcer
F. Hypertrophic gastropathy
G. Linitis plastica
H. Lymphoma
I. Peptic ulcer, chronic
J. Polyps
K. Pyloric stenosis
L. Trichobezoar

_____   6. A 40-year-old woman complained of burning epigastric pain, which usually occurred 1–3 hours after a meal. The pain could be relieved with antacids or food. Recently, she had noticed "coffee-grounds" material in her stool. Gastroscopy revealed a bleeding mucosal defect in the duodenum, measuring 2 cm in diameter. Biopsy showed that the lesion lacked mucosal lining cells and was composed of amorphous cellular detritus and neutrophils.

_____   7. A 45-year-old man complained of heartburn. A gastroscopic biopsy revealed chronic inflammation of the gastric mucosa. *Helicobacter pylori* organisms were found in the gastric foveolae. Treatment with antibiotics relieved his symptoms.

_____ **8.** A diffusely infiltrating carcinoma composed of signet ring cells had transformed the stomach into a "leather bottle"-like structure.

_____ **9.** A 50-year-old woman who suffered from rheumatoid arthritis complained of weakness and easy fatigability. Her stools had become black after she started taking a new nonsteroidal anti-inflammatory drug. Gastroscopy revealed numerous superficial, bleeding, mucosal defects.

_____ **10.** A 60-year-old man complained of loss of appetite, nausea, weight loss, and weakness. He had upper abdominal pain that did not respond to antacids or H2-receptor antagonists. A crater-like ulcerated lesion was detected in the antrum during gastroscopy. A biopsy of the lesion was composed of atypical, irregular, glandlike structures infiltrating the stroma.

DIRECTIONS: Match each numbered statement with the most appropriate lettered item. Each lettered item can be used once, more than once, or not at all.

Neoplasms of the Small and Large Intestine, Anus, and Appendix

A. Adenocarcinoma
B. Anal zone carcinoma
C. Carcinoid tumor
D. GIST (gastrointestinal stromal tumor)
E. Kaposi sarcoma
F. Leiomyosarcoma
G. Lipoma
H. Lymphoma
I. Metastatic carcinoma
J. Mucinous cystadenoma
K. Polyp, hamartomatous
L. Polyp, hyperplastic
M. Polyp, inflammatory
N. Polyp, lymphoid
O. Squamous cell carcinoma
P. Tubular adenoma
Q. Villous adenoma

_____ **11.** A small, raised, mucosal nodule of the colon, measuring 0.5 cm., is composed of crypts that have a serrated ("saw-toothed") appearance. It is lined by goblet cells and absorptive cells showing no signs of nuclear atypia.

_____ **12.** A small submucosal nodule in the ileum, measuring 1 cm in diameter, is composed of nests of cells, with round, uniform-sized nuclei and moderate amounts of cytoplasm. By electron micoscopy the cytoplasm contains neuroendocrine granules.

_____ **13.** A 2-cm nodule was passed in the bloody stool by a 5-year-old child. Histologically, the mass was composed of epithelial lined tubules filled with mucus.

_____ **14.** A "napkin ringlike" tumor circumferentially narrowed the rectum. Histologically, it was composed of irregular, glandlike structures, which were lined by hyperchromatic atypical cells.

_____ **15.** Multiple tumor nodules on the serosa of the small intestine.

DIRECTIONS: Choose the one best answer.

_____ **16.** Traction diverticula of the esophagus are typically found in the
A. pharyngo-esophageal junction.
B. upper third of the esophagus.
C. midportion of the esophagus.
D. lower third of the esophagus.
E. esophagogastric junction.

_____ **17.** Barrett esophagus is lined by epithelium that is histologically classified as
A. squamous.
B. glandular.
C. transitional.
D. stratified.
E. neuroepithelial.

_____ **18.** What is the most common cause of esophagitis?
A. Virus
B. Fungus
C. Bacteria
D. Immune factors
E. Gastric juice

_____ **19.** Multiple unrelenting ulcers of the stomach that are unresponsive to anti-ulcer therapy may be caused by tumors usually located in the
A. esophagus.
B. antrum of the stomach.
C. fundus of the stomach.
D. duodenum.
E. pancreas.

_____ **20.** What is the most common complication of peptic ulcer?
A. Bleeding
B. Stenosis
C. Perforation
D. Peritonitis
E. Malignant transformation

_____ 21. All the following statements about gastric lymphoma are true *except*
A. it is the most common form of extranodal lymphoma.
B. it accounts for about 20% of all extranodal lymphomas.
C. it has a worse prognosis than gastric carcinoma.
D. it presents with symptoms indistinguishable from those of carcinoma.
E. the diagnosis is established by gastric biopsy.

_____ 22. Toxigenic *E. coli* provokes diarrhea by
A. invading the mucosa of ileum.
B. invading the mucosa of colon.
C. stimulating transmucosal transport of fluid into the lumen of the intestine.
D. causing ulceration.
E. destroying Peyer's patches.

_____ 23. Diarrhea in infants under the age of 2 years is most often caused by
A. rotavirus.
B. cytomegalovirus.
C. *Yersinia jejuni.*
D. *Shigella dysenteriae.*
E. *Salmonella typhi.*

_____ 24. Transmural hemorrhagic infarcts occur most often in the
A. duodenum.
B. jejunum and ileum.
C. appendix.
D. cecum.
E. distal colon.

_____ 25. Diarrhea, episodic flushing, bronchospasm, and cardiac valve disease are typically caused by tumors classified as
A. adenocarcinoma.
B. leiomyosarcoma.
C. carcinoid.
D. lymphoma.
E. mesothelioma.

_____ 26. Hirschsprung disease (congenital megacolon) is a disorder involving the development of
A. nerves.
B. smooth muscle.
C. peritoneum.
D. blood vessels.
E. mucosa.

_____ 27. Patients with ulcerative colitis are at a higher risk than those with Crohn disease for developing
A. extraintestinal complications.
B. transmural inflammation.
C. cancer.
D. fistula.
E. stenosis.

_____ 28. Which colonic polyps are most likely to bleed?
    A. Hyperplastic polyp
    B. Peutz-Jeghers polyp
    C. Lymphoid polyp
    D. Tubular adenoma
    E. Villous adenoma

_____ 29. Squamous cell carcinoma typically originates in the
    A. ileum.
    B. cecum.
    C. transverse colon.
    D. rectum.
    E. anus.

_____ 30. Spontaneous bacterial peritonitis in school-aged children is typically a complication of
    A. nephrotic syndrome.
    B. sprue.
    C. meconium ileus.
    D. Hirschsprung disease.
    E. diverticulosis.

Answers

1. **The answer is A.** *Achalasia* of the esophagus is a functional cause of dysphagia (difficult swallowing), which is related to the failure of the LES
to relax. In primary achalasia the cause remains unknown. Secondary
achalasia can be a manifestation of Chagas disease, in which the ganglion cells regulating esophageal contraction are destroyed by *Trypanosoma cruzi.*

2. **The answer is P.** *Webs* are mucosal folds in the esophagus of some persons with dysphagia. Most often they appear in the upper esophagus.
They were previously often associated with Plummer-Vinson syndrome,
which is rare today. Webs differ from rings, which are thicker and contain smooth muscle. Lower esophageal rings are called Schatzki rings;
they are lined on the upper surface by squamous epithelium and on the
lower surface by columnar epithelium.

3. **The answer is B.** *Adenocarcinoma* of the esophagus is a malignant tumor
that commonly originates in the glandular metaplasia of Barret esophagus. It typically occurs in the lower third of the esophagus.

4. **The answer is H.** *Infectious esophagitis* usually develops in debiltated or
immunosuppressed persons and is most often caused by fungi or
viruses. In this case esophagitis was most likely caused by herpes simplex virus, type 1.

5. **The answer is K.** *Reflux esophagitis* is related to the entry of gastric juices
into the esophagus. It is most commonly associated with hiatal hernia
and various conditions that cause insufficiency of the lower esophageal
sphincter (e.g., alcoholism). Histologically, there is evidence of chronic
inflammation and reactive changes in the epithelium and the underlying
stroma.

6. **The answer is I.** *Peptic ulcer* is a localized defect of the mucosa of the stomach or duodenum, which tends to bleed and cause melena ("coffee grounds–like" black stools). Melena results from the action of hydrochloric acid upon hemoglobin in the stools.

7. **The answer is D.** *Chronic gastritis type B* is caused by *Helicobacter pylori*. By contrast, type A gastritis is autoimmune and is associated with vitamin B-12 deficiency and pernicious anemia.

8. **The answer is G.** *Linitis plastica* is a term used for gastric carcinoma that diffusely infiltrates all layers of the stomach, imparting a "leather bottle–like" appearance.

9. **The answer is A.** *Acute erosive gastritis* typically results from the intake of aspirin or nonsteroidal anti-inflammatory drugs, which cause bleeding from superficial mucosal defects (erosions).

10. **The answer is B.** *Adenocarcinoma* of the stomach is a tumor that most often presents as an ulcerated, indurated, mucosal mass, described as "craterlike." Histologically, it is indistinguishable from adenocarcinoma in other sites.

11. **The answer is L.** *Hyperplastic polyps* are inuocuous, small, mucosal nodules composed of well-differentiated goblet and absorptive cells, similar to those in the normal colon.

12. **The answer is C.** *Carcinoid tumors* are low-grade malignant neoplasms composed of neuroendocrine cells, which usually show considerable nuclear uniformity.

13. **The answer is K.** *Hamartomatous polyps*, also known as retention or juvenile polyps, are typically found in the rectum of children under the age of 10 years. They may undergo self-amputation and pass in the stool.

14. **The answer is A.** *Adenocarcinoma* of the rectum or sigmoid colon often presents as a circumferential mass narrowing the intestinal lumen.

15. **The answer is I.** *Metastatic carcinoma* to the abdomen often presents in the form of multiple serosal nodules and ascites that contains malignant cells.

16. **The answer is C.** Diverticula of the *midportion* of the esophagus have been traditionally called "traction diverticula" because their triangular shape, with a broad base toward the lumen, suggests that the wall has been retracted by an external force (e.g., adhesions to tuberculous lymph nodes). Such an etiology is uncommon today. Owing to their shape, these diverticula do not retain food and are mostly asymptomatic. By contrast, "epiphrenic diverticula" are often associated with disturbances of esophageal motility and reflux esophagitis.

17. **The answer is B.** Barrett epithelium is a patch of *glandular epithelium* that replaces the normal squamous epithelium of the esophagus in persons who suffer from prolonged reflux esophagitis. In most instances, reflux is caused by incompetence of the lower esophageal sphincter. Since columnar epithelium of Barrett esophagus is more resistant to peptic juices, it seems to be an adaptive metaplasia, which limits the adverse effects of gastric reflux.

18. **The answer is E.** Reflux esophagitis caused by *gastric juice* is a common condition and is the most frequent cause of chronic inflammation in the

esophagus. Bacterial infections in otherwise healthy persons are unusual because the esophageal mucosa is resistant to bacterial invasion. Fungal esophagitis and that caused by herpesvirus in immunosuppressed persons are characterized by plaquelike lesions of pseudomembranous esophagitis.

19. **The answer is E.** Gastrin-producing neuroendocrine tumors usually arise in the *pancreas*; by secreting gastrin they may produce the Zollinger-Ellison syndrome, characterized by unrelenting peptic ulceration in the stomach or duodenum, or even in the proximal jejunum.

20. **The answer is A.** *Bleeding* is the most common complication of peptic ulcer, occurring in about 20% of patients. Chronic blood loss due to occult bleeding is often a feature of peptic ulcers, whereas massive bleeding occurs less often. Perforation is uncommon, but when it occurs it is more likely to be located in the duodenum. It is more likely to be fatal in patients with gastric ulcers.

21. **The answer is C.** Gastric lymphoma is the most common form of extranodal lymphoma, comprising 20% of such tumors. It has a considerably *better prognosis* than gastric carcinoma (45% 5-year survival). The clinical symptoms are nonspecific and indistinguishable from those of carcinoma. The diagnosis is established by gastric biopsy.

22. **The answer is C.** Toxigenic bacteria such as certain strains of *E. coli* provoke diarrhea by stimulating *transmucosal transport of fluids* into the lumen. Altered absorption and increased peristalsis are considered to be less important. Cholera, another toxigenic microorganism, does not invade or destroy the intestinal mucosa. By contrast, *Salmonella typhi* invades the intestine and multiplies in the lymphoid follicles of the wall. The mucosa overlying the infected lymphoid tissue, especially over Peyer's patches, undergoes necrosis, with the subsequent formation of ulcers.

23. **The answer is A.** *Rotavirus* is the most common cause of infantile diarrhea and can be demonstrated in duodenal biopsy specimens in half the cases of acute diarrhea in hospitalized children under the age of 2 years.

24. **The answer is B.** The *small intestine* is more likely to suffer transmural hemorrhagic infarction than the large intestine. The inferior mesenteric artery, which supplies blood to the colon, is a less common site for embolization than the superior mesenteric artery, because of the smaller size of the latter and its oblique origin from the aorta. The richer collateral circulation in the large intestine provides another compensatory mechanism. Venous thrombosis predominantly involves the small intestine and almost invariably involves the superior mesenteric vein.

25. **The answer is C.** The most prominent findings in the *carcinoid syndrome* are diarrhea, episodic flushing, bronchospasm, and cardiac valvular disease. These symptoms are produced by serotonin and perhaps other vasoactive amines and their metabolites, which are released into the systemic circulation from metastatic tumors in the liver or some other site. If the carcinoid tumor is limited to the intestine, vasoactive substances are released into the portal circulation and, upon reaching the liver, are inactivated. Because of the local effects of substances released from the neuroendocrine tumor cells in the intestine, diarrhea may be a symptom of localized tumors that have not spread beyond the intestine.

26. **The answer is A.** Hirschsprung disease results from a congenital defect in the *innervation* of the large intestine, usually in the rectum. Typically, the ganglion cells in a portion of the colon do not develop properly and the aganglionic segment undergoes permanent contraction. Marked dilatation of the colon occurs proximal to the stenotic rectum, with clinical signs of intestinal obstruction. A biopsy of the aganglionic rectum can be diagnostic, but only if the specimen includes the muscularis, where the ganglion cells normally reside.

27. **The answer is C.** Ulcerative colitis and Crohn disease share many common features. Extraintestinal systemic symptoms occur in both diseases. *Cancer* may develop in the large intestine with both disorders, although the risk is *three times higher* for patients with ulcerative colitis.

28. **The answer is E.** All intestinal polyps can bleed, but the broad-based *villous tumors* are more easily traumatized than the smaller, pedunculated tubular adenomas.

29. **The answer is E.** Whereas cancers of the large intestine are mostly adenocarcinomas, squamous cell carcinoma arises in the *anal canal*.

30. **The answer is A.** Most cases of peritonitis are caused by bacteria that enter the abdominal cavity from a perforated viscus or through an abdominal wound. However, bacterial peritonitis occurs in children without an obvious perforation. Most of these patients have the *nephrotic syndrome* and a systemic infection that seeds the ascitic fluid with bacteria. In adults, spontaneous bacterial peritonitis is a feared complication of cirrhosis.

Chapter 14

The Liver and Biliary System

Questions

DIRECTIONS: Match each numbered statement with the most appropriate lettered item. Each lettered item can be used once, more than once, or not at all.

Liver Diseases

A. Abscess of the liver
B. Alcoholic hepatitis
C. Alpha-1-antitrypsin deficiency
D. Autoimmune hepatitis
E. Budd-Chiari syndrome
F. Cholangitis
G. Cholecystitis
H. Cholelithiasis
I. Cholestatic jaundice
J. Cirrhosis
K. Drug-induced hepatitis
L. Fatty liver
M. Gilbert syndrome
N. Hemolytic jaundice
O. Hereditary hemochromatosis
P. Primary biliary cirrhosis
Q. Primary sclerosing cholangitis
R. Viral hepatitis, acute
S. Viral hepatitis, chronic
T. Wilson disease

_____ **1.** An 18-year-old college freshman noticed yellow discoloration of his skin and sclerae. He had no other symptoms. An elevated bilirubin level (7 mg/dL), mostly in unconjugated form, was the only laboratory abnormality. His brother was found to have

hyperbilirubinemia as well. Jaundice disappeared spontaneously.

_____ 2. A 3-day-old neonate was found to be extremely yellow. No
underlying disease was found, and the mother was assured that
the jaundice would disappear without treatment.

_____ 3. A 70-year-old man was diagnosed with carcinoma of the pancreas and developed jaundice. The serum bilirubin was elevated
(25 mg/dL), most of it conjugated.

_____ 4. A 20-year-old woman returned from vacationing in Mexico complaining of mild fever, malaise, and loss of appetite. A week later
she noticed that her eyes became yellow and her urine turned
brown. Laboratory tests disclosed hyperbilirubinemia and elevated serum levels of alanine aminotransferase, and aspartate
aminotransferase, but normal albumin and globulin levels. A test
for hepatitis virus A(HAV) infection disclosed IgM-anti-HAV in
a titer of 1:256 but no IgG-anti-HAV.

_____ 5. A 30-year-old man complained of tiredness and occasional fever.
He also noticed yellow sclerae, tenderness below the right costal
margin, and dark urine. Liver function tests were abnormal. A
liver biopsy revealed expansion of the portal tracts by lymphocytic infiltrates, which also penetrated across the limiting plate
into the lobule and surrounded groups of hepatocytes. Serologic
tests revealed antibodies to hepatitis B core of the IgG type (IgG
anti-HBcAg). HBsAg and HBeAg were also present, but there
were no antibodies to either HBsAg or HBeAg.

_____ 6. A 20-year-old woman developed jaundice. She also noticed that
her menses had ceased and that her mouth was dry. Laboratory
tests disclosed no signs of viral hepatitis. There was hypergammaglobulinemia (5.5 g/dL), and the antinuclear antibody
(ANA), and anti–smooth muscle antibody (ASMA) titers were
highly elevated. Liver biopsy disclosed intralobular and peripor-
tal inflammatory cell infiltrates, composed of lymphocytes and
plasma cells.

DIRECTIONS: Match each numbered statement with the most appropriate
lettered item. Each lettered item can be used once, more than once, or not
at all.

Tumors of Hepatobiliary Tract

A. Carcinoma of common bile duct
B. Carcinoma of the gall bladder
C. Cholangiocarcinoma
D. Hemangiosarcoma
E. Hepatoblastoma
F. Hepatocellular adenoma
G. Hepatocellular carcinoma
H. Metastatic carcinoma

_____ **7.** A 2-cm adenocarcinoma located at the ampulla of Vater.

_____ **8.** Squamous cell carcinoma locally invading the gallbladder wall and extending into the liver.

_____ **9.** Primary liver tumor composed of polygonal tumor cells arranged in cords and resembling normal hepatocytes but showing nuclear pleomorphism and hyperchromasia. It was accompanied by elevation of serum alphafetoprotein.

_____ **10.** Adenocarcinoma in a native of China infected with *Opistorchis sinensis*.

_____ **11.** Multiple circumscribed, grayish-white nodules involving both lobes of the liver.

DIRECTIONS: Choose the one best answer.

_____ **12.** Liver biopsy performed on a 65-year-old jaundiced man revealed severe cholestasis, feathery degeneration of hepatocytes, and bile lakes. These findings are most consistent with the diagnosis of
A. cirrhosis.
B. extrahepatic biliary obstruction.
C. Gilbert disease.
D. viral hepatitis.
E. Budd-Chiari syndrome.

_____ **13.** In hepatorenal syndrome the kidney biopsy would show
A. no histologic changes.
B. focal necrosis of glomerular capillaries.
C. proliferative glomerulonephritis.
D. interstitial nephritis.
E. renal tubular necrosis.

_____ **14.** Coagulation disturbances encountered in chronic liver disease typically include deficiencies of all the following coagulation factors *except*
A. Factor I (fibrinogen).
B. Factor II (prothrombin).
C. Factor VII.
D. Factor VIII.
E. von Willebrand factor.

_____ **15.** A patient with advanced cirrhosis is prone to show
A. hypoalbuminemia.
B. thrombocytosis.
C. hypogammaglobulinemia.
D. hirsutism.
E. increased serum testosterone in blood.

_____ **16.** Fulminant hepatic failure is most often caused by which hepatitis virus?
A. A
B. B
C. C
D. D
E. E

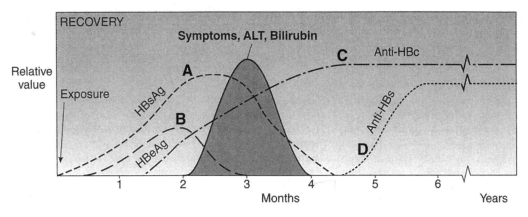

FIGURE 14-1.   VIRUSOLOGIC AND SEROLOGIC FINDINGS IN VIRAL HEPATITIS **B**.

DIRECTIONS: Match the following numbered words or phrases with the most appropriate lettered curve in Figure 14-1. Each lettered curve can be used once, more than once, or not at all.

_A_   **17.** First serologic evidence of infection
_C_   **18.** Antibodies that do not terminate the disease
_D_   **19.** Antibodies that confer immunity
_B_   **20.** Persistence that indicates chronic infectivity
_D_   **21.** Does not appear in chronic carriers

DIRECTIONS: Choose the one best answer.

_B_   **22.** A chronic alcoholic was found by biopsy to have fatty liver. If he stops drinking, his liver will most likely
   A. remain fatty.
   B. revert to normal.
   C. become fibrotic.
   D. progress to alcoholic hepatitis.
   E. progress to alcoholic cirrhosis.

_E_   **23.** Mallory bodies are associated with
   A. viral hepatitis A.
   B. viral hepatitis B.
   C. viral hepatitis C.
   D. viral hepatitis E.
   E. alcoholic hepatitis.

_A_   **24.** Which of the following diseases is characterized by destruction of intrahepatic bile ducts?
   A. Primary biliary cirrhosis
   B. Secondary biliary cirrhosis
   C. Gilbert disease
   D. Alpha-1-antitrypsin deficiency
   E. Wilson disease

25. In hereditary hemochromatosis Kupffer cells, hepatocytes and bile ducts in the liver contain increased amounts of
   A. copper.
   B. iron.
   C. zinc.
   D. hemoglobin.
   E. ceruloplasmin.

26. Kayser-Fleischer rings in the eyes and extrapyramidal neurologic symptoms are typical of
   A. hemosiderosis.
   B. hereditary hemochromatosis.
   C. Wilson disease.
   D. Crigler-Najjar syndrome.
   E. Indian childhood cirrhosis.

27. Posthepatic portal hypertension is most likely associated with
   A. primary biliary cirrhosis.
   B. secondary biliary cirrhosis.
   C. portal vein thrombosis.
   D. polycythemia vera.
   E. intrahepatic cholestasis.

28. Liver biopsy in Reye syndrome shows
   A. fibrosis.
   B. cirrhosis.
   C. steatosis.
   D. hemosiderosis.
   E. thrombosis.

29. All the following are predisposing factors for cholelithiasis and cholecystitis *except*
   A. multiparity.
   B. female sex.
   C. obesity.
   D. diabetes.
   E. uremia.

30. The incidence of pigment stones is increased in association with
   A. diabetes.
   B. atherosclerosis.
   C. hypercholesterolemia.
   D. aplastic anemia.
   E. sickle cell disease.

Answers

1. The answer is M. *Gilbert disease* is a familial disease presenting as recurrent unconjugated hyperbilirubinemia. Except for episodes of jaundice these patients are asymptomatic.

2. The answer is N. *Hemolytic jaundice* owing to the postpartum destruction of red blood cells carrying fetal hemoglobin occurs when there is inadequate conjugation in hepatocytes (due to low activity of UDP-glucuronyltransferase). This situation leads to physiologic unconjugated hyperbilirubinemia.

3. **The answer is I.** Obstruction of the common bile duct by pancreatic cancer leads to *cholestatic jaundice*. The blood contains increased amounts of conjugated bilirubin.

4. **The answer is R.** *Viral hepatitis* caused by HAV is an acute, self-limited disease. IgM-anti-HAV is the first serologic sign of HAV infection, and its titers peak during the first week of clinical disease. Titers of IgG-anti-HAV peak approximately 1 month after the onset of disease. IgM becomes undetectable after 3–6 months, whereas IgG titers remain high for years.

5. **The answer is S.** *Chronic hepatitis* B presents with nonspecific clinical symptoms and sometimes jaundice. The diagnosis depends on laboratory and biopsy findings.

6. **The answer is D.** *Autoimmune hepatitis* typically affects young women but may occur in older women and men as well. It is often accompanied by other autoimmune diseases (e.g., Sjögren disease, or SLE). Hypergammaglobulinemia and antibodies to nuclear antigens (ANA) or smooth muscle antigens (SMA) are typical. The disease responds well to corticosteroids.

7. **The answer is A.** *Adenocarcinoma of the common bile duct*, which may arise at the ampulla of Vater, causes jaundice early in the course of the disease.

8. **The answer is B.** *Carcinoma of the gallbladder* most often presents as adenocarcinoma, but in 10% of cases it is a squamous cell carcinoma. These tumors originate from foci of squamous metaplasia that occur in chronic cholecystitis associated with gallstones.

9. **The answer is G.** *Hepatocellular carcinoma* is a primary liver tumor composed of neoplastic hepatocytes. The tumor cells typically secrete AFP into the blood, thereby providing a serologic marker for hepatocellular carcinoma.

10. **The answer is C.** *Cholangiocarcinoma* is an adenocarcinoma originating from intraheptic bile ducts. Ca of common ducts may also be more common. These tumors occur at an increased frequency in persons infected with liver fluke cholestasis sinensis.

11. **The answer is H.** *Metastatic carcinoma* to the liver typically presents as multiple nodules.

12. **The answer is B.** Feathery degeneration and bile lakes are caused by the toxic effect of bile pigment on liver cells and are features of *chronic biliary obstruction*. *Feathery degeneration* refers to hydropic vacuolization of liver cells, with the intracellular accumulation of bile pigment. It is reversible, in contrast to *bile lakes*, a term used to denote the necrosis of groups of bile-containing liver cells and the extracellular accumulation of bile.

13. **The answer is A.** The hepatorenal syndrome represents functional renal failure in patients with hepatic failure. Histologically, the kidney *appears normal* and shows no evidence of toxic tubular necrosis. Renal failure is due to hypoperfusion of the kidneys, mediated by various hormones and vasoactive substances. These substances accumulate in the blood because the liver does not efficiently remove them from the circulation.

Following surgical removal of the diseased liver and liver transplantation, the kidneys may resume normal function. Similarly, the kidneys from a patient in hepatic coma may be transplanted into another person and function normally.

14. **The answer is E.** *Fibrinogen, prothrombin, factor VII, and factor VIII* are all produced in the liver. A prolonged prothrombin time in these patients correlates best with low plasma concentrations of factor VII. Von Willebrand factor is produced by endothelial cells and platelets.

15. **The answer is A.** Patients with cirrhosis have *hypoalbuminemia* because of impaired protein synthesis by hepatocytes.

16. **The answer is B.** Overall, fulminant hepatic failure is a rare outcome of acute viral hepatitis, but it is a well-recognized feature of *hepatitis B*. It occurs rarely with hepatitis C, and only exceptionally with hepatitis A.

17. **The answer is A.** *Surface antigen* (HBsAg) in the serum provides the first evidence of infection and disappears over a period of 3 to 5 months. It is present in the serum in both asymptomatic carriers and those with chronic active hepatitis.

18. **The answer is C.** *Antibodies to the core antigen* (anti-HBcAg) appear after a few weeks in all patients infected with hepatitis B virus. They do not confer immunity but are used as a serologic marker of previous infection.

19. **The answer is D.** *Antibodies to the surface antigen* (anti-HBsAg) confer immunity.

20. **The answer is B.** In the course of acute hepatitis B, the *e antigen* (HBeAg) appears after HBsAg but disappears earlier in patients who recover without incident. The presence of HBeAg marks the period of highest infectivity. The persistence of HBeAg is usually associated with chronic hepatitis and indicates continued infectivity.

21. **The answer is D.** *Antibodies to HBsAg* are not present in chronic carriers. This lack is presumably responsible for the inability to clear the virus.

22. **The answer is A.** Upon cessation of alcohol abuse, the fatty liver *reverts to normal*.

23. **The answer is E.** Mallory bodies are a common finding in *alcoholic hepatitis*. Although they are not pathognomonic of this condition, their presence is a useful histologic finding for diagnosing alcoholic liver injury. Similar cytoplasmic hyaline bodies can be seen in other conditions, including Wilson disease and hepatocellular carcinoma, as well as after jejunoileal bypass surgery for morbid obesity.

24. **The answer is A.** *Primary biliary cirrhosis* is thought to be an autoimmune disease, and, like most other autoimmune disorders, it occurs more often in women than in men. The disease typically presents with chronic destruction of bile ducts in the portal tracts. Patients with primary biliary cirrhosis have various autoantibodies, but 90% display antimitochondrial antibodies. Antimitochondrial antibodies are not thought to be involved in the pathogenesis of primary biliary cirrhosis, but they are useful for the diagnosis of the disease.

25. **The answer is B.** Hemochromatosis is characterized by the accumulation of *iron* in the liver and other organs. Wilson disease is marked by the deposition of copper.

26. **The answer is C.** Ocular lesions, the so-called Kayser-Fleischer ring, and extrapyramidal neurologic symptoms related to degenerative changes in the corpus striatum are common in *Wilson disease*.

27. **The answer is D.** Posthepatic portal hypertension is caused by obstruction of venous outflow from the liver by thrombi (Budd-Chiari syndrome) or tumors. Intrahepatic venous thrombosis may be associated with increased blood viscosity, as in *polycythemia vera* or hypercoagulability states. However, in more one than half the cases, the cause of Budd-Chiari syndrome is not known.

28. **The answer is C.** Reye syndrome occurs most often in small children after an acute febrile illness that has been treated with aspirin. It presents with hepatic failure and encephalopathy, but the pathogenesis of this syndrome and its relation to aspirin are not understood. The liver biopsy consistently shows microvesicular *steatosis* (fatty change). Electron microscopy reveals changes in liver mitochondria.

29. **The answer is E.** Cholelithiasis and cholecystitis are closely related disorders that occur more often in women than in men and have comparable predisposing factors, including obesity, diabetes, and multiparity. Gallstones are not a complication of *uremia*.

30. **The answer is E.** Hemolysis that occurs in patients with *sickle cell disease* generates excess bilirubin, which predisposes to pigment stone formation.

The Pancreas

Questions

DIRECTIONS: Match each numbered statement with the most appropriate lettered item. Each lettered item can be used once, more than once, or not at all.

Nonneoplastic Diseases of the Pancreas

A. Aberrant pancreas
B. Acute hemorrhagic pancreatitis
C. Acute interstitial pancreatitis
D. Annular pancreas
E. Chronic pancreatitis
F. Pancreas divisum
G. Pancreatic pseudocyst
H. Retention cyst

1. A 50-year-old man with a 10-year history of alcohol abuse presented to the emergency room complaining of severe pain in his upper abdomen for the last 12 hours. The pain radiated to the back and was associated with an urge to vomit. He had tachycardia, tachypnea, and hypotension. There was no ascites or guarding of abdominal muscles. Serum amylase was elevated five times over the normal value.

2. A 45-year-old chronic alcoholic complained of recurrent attacks of pain that would develop gradually over a few hours after he had consumed his evening libations. The pain radiated into his back and could be relieved upon leaning forward. He also complained of loose, bulky, greasy stools and bouts of diarrhea. X-ray revealed abdominal calcifications.

3. A 50-year-old woman was hospitalized 6 weeks after a bout of acute abdominal pain and elevated levels of serum amylase and lipase. She complained of cramps after meals and a tendency to regurgitate food. Physical examination revealed jaundice, and a CAT scan disclosed an inhomogeneous pancreatic mass. An ultrasound examination suggested that it might be hollow.

_____ 4. A neonate experienced bouts of vomiting and could not be fed adequately. Gastroscopy and x-ray examination disclosed marked narrowing of the duodenum, owing to a mass encircling the midportion of the duodenum.

DIRECTIONS: Match each numbered statement with the most appropriate lettered item. Each lettered item can be used once, more than once, or not at all.

Tumors of the Pancreas

A. Adenocarcinoma
B. Carcinoid
C. Cystadenoma
D. Gastrinoma
E. Glucagonoma
F. Insulinoma
G. Pancreatic polypeptide-secreting tumor
H. Somatostatinoma
I. VIPoma

_____ 5. Most common tumor of the pancreas
_____ 6. The most common cause of obstructive jaundice
_____ 7. Cause of Trousseau syndrome
_____ 8. Most common pancreatic islet cell tumor
_____ 9. Necrotizing erythematous rash of the lower body
_____ 10. Attacks of sweating, nervousness, and hunger
_____ 11. Watery diarrhea, hypokalemia, and hypochlorhydria
_____ 12. Intractable peptic ulcer

DIRECTIONS: Match the following numbered words or phrases with the most appropriate lettered part of Figure 15-1. Each lettered part can be used once, more than once, or not at all.

_____ 13. Lesion typically associated with pain radiating into the back
_____ 14. Histologic appearance of an endocrine tumor
_____ 15. Histologic appearance of a gastrin-producing tumor
_____ 16. Neuroendocrine granules

A n s w e r s

1. **The answer is B.** *Acute hemorrhagic pancreatitis* typically presents with upper abdominal pain of sudden onset, often accompanied by signs of shock, such as tachypnea, tachycardia, and hypotension. Radiologic studies are helpful in visualizing the edematous and hemorrhagic enlargement of the pancreas.

2. **The answer is E.** *Chronic pancreatitis* is characterized by upper abdominal pain that evolves gradually over several hours after a heavy meal or

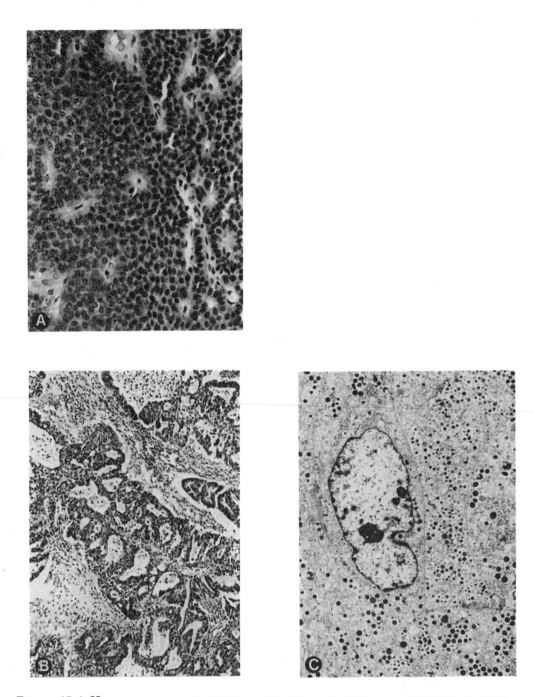

FIGURE 15-1. HISTOLOGIC AND ELECTRON MICROSCOPIC FEATURES OF PANCREATIC TUMORS.

a drinking episode. X-rays usually disclose specks of calcification and pancreatic intraductal calculi. Pancreatic insufficiency results in steatorrhea or diarrhea. Long-lasting disease is accompanied by signs of malabsorption and nutritional deficiency, such as weight loss, anemia, osteomalacia, and a tendency to bleed.

3. **The answer is G.** *Pancreatic pseudocyst* is a complication of acute hemorrhagic pancreatitis, in which the necrotic pancreatic tissue is liquefied through the action of pancreatic enzymes, including peptidases, lipase, and amylase. The necrotic tissue becomes encapsulated by granulation tissue, which develops into a fibrous capsule. Pseudocyst may act as a mass and obstruct the duodenum or the bile duct.

4. **The answer is D.** *Annular pancreas*, a developmental anomaly, may encircle the duodenum and cause duodenal obstruction.

5. **The answer is A.** *Adenocarcinoma* is the most common pancreatic neoplasm and one of the most common malignant tumors. Although it accounts for only 3% of all cancers in the United States, it is the fifth leading cause of death from cancer.

6. **The answer is A.** Owing to their location in the head of the pancreas, *adenocarcinomas* often present with jaundice, caused by the obstruction of the common bile duct. Painless dilation of the gallbladder accompanied by jaundice is termed *Courvoisier sign* and may be the first evidence of pancreatic cancer.

7. **The answer is A.** Trousseau syndrome, or migratory thrombophlebitis, may accompany *adenocarcinoma* of the pancreas. It is thought that the tumor releases thrombogenic substances into the circulation, notably serine proteases, that initiate the coagulation cascade and cause disseminated venous thrombosis.

8. **The answer is F.** *Insulinoma* is the most common islet cell tumor.

9. **The answer is E.** Necrotizing migratory erythema develops in association with the hypersecretion of glucagon by α-cell-containing tumors (glucagonomas). These patients also have mild diabetes and anemia.

10. **The answer is F.** *Insulinomas* secrete insulin, which in turn causes hypoglycemia. The symptoms of hypoglycemia include hunger, sweating, irritability, epileptic seizures, and coma. The infusion of glucose alleviates the symptoms.

11. **The answer is I.** Intractable diarrhea, hypokalemia, and low levels of chloride in gastric juice comprise the syndrome of "pancreatic cholera." This disorder is secondary to the secretion of *vasoactive intestinal polypeptide* (VIP) by an islet cell tumor. VIP stimulates adenylyl cyclase activity, which in turn leads to the production of large amounts of cAMP. The latter causes increased secretion of potassium and water into the intestinal lumen. The ensuing diarrhea results in a loss of water, amounting to as much as 5 L/day.

12. **The answer is D.** Intractable peptic ulcers, multiple ulcers, and ulcers in atypical locations may be part of the Zollinger-Ellison syndrome and are caused by *gastrinomas*. Gastrinomas are most often located in the pancreas, but they may be found in other parts of the gastrointestinal tract, notably the duodenum. Gastrinoma is the second most common endocrine tumor of the pancreas.

13. **The answer is B.** Figure 15-1B illustrates an *adenocarcinoma*, the prototype of a malignant tumor originating from the exocrine ducts. The desmoplastic (fibrosing) reaction is typical of pancreatic adenocarcinoma.

14. **The answer is A.** Figure 15-1A illustrates the characteristic histologic appearance of *endocrine tumors* of the pancreas. The cells have a uniform appearance, with round nuclei and a moderate amount of cytoplasm. They form ribbons, strands, and small groups, intermixed with a capillary network.

15. **The answer is A.** Figure 15-1A is representative of all endocrine tumors, including the *gastrin-producing tumor* illustrated here.

16. **The answer is C.** Figure 15-1C shows the electron microscopic appearance of a *gastrinoma*. The cytoplasm contains dense, membrane-bound, neuroendocrine granules, which show a clear halo between the central dense core and the limiting membrane.

Chapter 16

The Kidney

Questions

DIRECTIONS: Match each numbered statement with the most appropriate lettered item. Each lettered item can be used once, more than once, or not at all.

Glomerular Disease

    A. Acute glomerulonephritis
    B. Alport syndrome
    C. Amyloidosis
    D. Chronic glomerulonephritis
    E. Crescentic glomerulonephritis
    F. Diffuse proliferative glomerulonephritis
    G. Focal proliferative glomerulonephritis
    H. Focal necrotizing glomerulonephritis
    I. Focal segmental glomerulosclerosis
    J. Membranoproliferative glomerulonephritis, type I
    K. Membranoproliferative glomerulonephritis, type II
    L. Membranous nephropathy
    M. Minimal change disease (lipoid nephrosis)
    N. Nodular or diffuse diabetic glomerulosclerosis

_____ 1. Oliguria, proteinuria, hematuria, and generalized edema developed in a 6-year-old boy 2 weeks after a severe throat infection, after which a renal biopsy was performed. The glomeruli showed hypercellularity, reflecting endothelial and mesangial cell proliferation, and infiltrates of neutrophils and macrophages.

_____ 2. Mild proteinuria and microscopic hematuria were found in a 25-year-old man. In the renal biopsy, some glomeruli showed mesangial proliferation, with mesangial deposits of IgA. The clinician told the patient that this is the most common form of glomerular disease and that in most cases it has a good prognosis. No treatment was given.

_____ 3. Nephrotic syndrome developed in a 60-year-old man with multiple myeloma.

_____ 4. Nephrotic syndrome developed in a man who had chronic purulent bronchiectasis.

_____ 5. A man who had viral hepatitis B developed nephrotic syndrome. A renal biopsy showed thickening of the glomerular basement membranes, which contained granular deposits of immunoglobulins. Electron microscopy showed that the deposits were subepithelial.

_____ 6. A biopsy diagnosis of Goodpasture syndrome was made 3 weeks after the onset of oliguria and hematuria.

_____ 7. Proteinuria in a drug addict prompted a renal biopsy, which disclosed obliteration of capillary loops in some of the glomeruli.

_____ 8. This most common secondary form of nephrotic syndrome in adults is also associated with glucosuria.

_____ 9. A 35-year-old woman developed Wegener granulomatosis. A renal biopsy showed no glomerular crescents, but the basement membranes of some glomeruli were ruptured and focally impregnated with fibrin.

_____ 10. Steroid responsive nephrotic syndrome was diagnosed in a 4-year-old child. Renal biopsy disclosed normal glomeruli.

_____ 11. Kimmelstiel-Wilson disease was diagnosed by renal biopsy in a diabetic man, who also had proteinuria.

_____ 12. This mild form of nephritis in systemic lupus erythematosus is marked by hypercellularity of some glomeruli.

_____ 13. In this most severe form of nephritis in systemic lupus erythematosus, more than 50% of the glomeruli appear hypercellular. They show mesangial and endocapillary proliferation, inflammatory cell infiltration, and "wire loop" formation.

DIRECTIONS: Choose the one best answer.

_____ 14. Acute renal failure secondary to cardiogenic shock is characterized by
A. oliguria.
B. polyuria.
C. hematuria.
D. proteinuria.
E. glycosuria.

_____ 15. Which of the following is a constant feature of nephrotic syndrome?
A. Oliguria
B. Polyuria
C. Hematuria
D. Proteinuria
E. Glycosuria

_____ **16.** Rapidly progressive glomerulonephritis is histologically charac-
terized by
A. endothelial cell proliferation
B. mesangial cell proliferation
C. formation of crescents in the urinary space
D. focal hyalinization of glomerular loops
E. wire loop formation

_____ **17.** Most ectopic kidneys are located
A. caudal to their expected location
B. cranial to their expected location
C. at the same side of the body as expected
D. on the contralateral side
E. in the anterior abdomen

_____ **18.** Which of the following congenital renal diseases is inherited as
an autosomal dominant trait?
A. Adult polycystic kidney disease
B. Infantile polycystic kidney disease
C. Medullary sponge kidney
D. Medullary cystic kidney disease complex
E. Cystic renal dysplasia

_____ **19.** Which systemic disease may produce glomerular changes indis-
tinguishable from those seen in membranous nephropathy?
A. Systemic sclerosis (scleroderma)
B. Systemic lupus erythematosus
C. Diabetes mellitus
D. Goodpasture syndrome
E. Wegener granulomatosis

_____ **20.** Acute pyelonephritis is most often caused by
A. immune complex deposition
B. viruses
C. Gram-negative bacteria
D. Gram-positive bacteria
E. mycobacteria

_____ **21.** Allergic drug-induced kidney disease presents most often in the
form of
A. crescentic glomerulonephritis
B. focal necrotizing glomerulonephritis
C. acute tubulointerstitial nephritis
D. chronic pyelonephritis
E. renal papillary necrosis

_____ **22.** Uric acid crystal deposits in the kidney are typically found in
patients treated for
A. angina pectoris
B. bronchopneumonia
C. acute cystitis
D. acute leukemia
E. rheumatoid arthritis

_____ **23.** Acute renal failure in pregnancy complicated by abruptio placentae is caused by
    A. crescentic glomerulonephritis
    B. necrotizing glomerulonephritis
    C. acute tubulointerstitial nephritis
    D. bilateral renal cortical necrosis
    E. renal papillary necrosis

_____ **24.** Fibrinoid necrosis of the renal arterioles is typically caused by
    A. benign hypertension related to arteriolonephrosclerosis
    B. malignant hypertension
    C. hemolytic uremic syndrome
    D. toxemia of pregnancy
    E. fibromuscular dysplasia

_____ **25.** Most renal stones in the United States are composed of
    A. calcium oxalate
    B. calcium phosphate
    C. magnesium ammonium phosphate
    D. uric acid
    E. cystine

_____ **26.** Most renal cell carcinomas originate from
    A. glomeruli
    B. tubules
    C. juxtaglomerular cells
    D. renal calices
    E. renal papillae

_____ **27.** A renal tumor of infancy composed of immature cells of the renal primordium or immature tubules is called
    A. Grawitz tumor
    B. Wilms tumor
    C. Ewing sarcoma
    D. metanephric adenoma
    E. angiomyolipoma

_____ **28.** Papillary carcinomas of the renal pelvis are histologically classified as
    A. squamous cell carcinoma
    B. transitional cell carcinoma
    C. small cell carcinoma
    D. basal cell carcinoma
    E. carcinosarcoma

Answers

1. **The answer is A.** *Acute glomerulonephritis* presents with typical nephritic signs and symptoms, which include oliguria, proteinuria, hematuria, and hypoproteinemia, the last leading to generalized edema. This immune complex-mediated disease typically develops after a streptococcal infection, most often involving the upper respiratory tract. Deposits of immune complexes in the glomeruli elicit an acute inflammatory response, and the affected glomeruli appear hypercellular,

owing to the proliferation of endothelial and mesangial cells and infiltrates of inflammatory cells.

2. **The answer is G.** *Focal proliferative glomerulonephritis* typically presents with pathologic changes in some glomeruli, whereas others remain normal. This group of diseases includes lupus nephritis, nephritis that accompanies several vasculitides, Henoch-Schönlein purpura and several other disorders. It also includes IgA nephropathy (Berger disease), which, as in this case, presents with mesangial deposits of IgA and mesangial cell proliferation.

3. **The answer is C.** *Amyloidosis* is a common complication of multiple myeloma. Deposits of AL amyloid, which is derived from the light chains of IgG, are characteristically found in the glomeruli but may also appear in the tubular basement membranes and in the walls of renal vessels. Renal amyloidosis usually presents as nephrotic syndrome.

4. **The answer is C.** *Amyloidosis* is a well-known complication of chronic suppurative disorders, such as chronic suppurative bronchiectasis or osteomyelitis. These conditions stimulate the production of amyloid from the serum amyloid A protein, an acute phase reactant secreted by the liver. Systemic amyloidosis under these conditions is characterized by deposits of amyloid fibrils in the blood vessels in many organs and is most often diagnosed in tissue obtained by rectal biopsy. The kidneys, liver, spleen, and adrenals are the most common organs involved. Nephrotic syndrome caused by deposition of SAA amyloid is clinically indistinguishable from that related to AL amyloid.

5. **The answer is L.** *Membranous nephropathy* is a complication of viral hepatitis B. In the early stages of infection, antibodies to viral proteins react with the antigen in the blood to form immune complexes. These deposit in the glomeruli, thereby altering the permeability of the glomerular basement membrane. The resulting proteinuria leads to hypoproteinemia, and generalized edema (i.e., clinically recognizable nephrotic syndrome). Morphologically, the glomerular basement membranes appear thickened, owing to massive deposition of immune complexes on the subepithelial side of the membranes, which evoke almost no inflammation.

6. **The answer is E.** *Crescentic glomerulonephritis* is the morphologic equivalent of the acute renal failure that develops in rapidly progressive glomerulonephritis of Goodpasture syndrome. This disease is mediated by antibodies to collagen type IV, which attack the glomerular basement membrane. This effect leads to rupture of the GBM and extravasation of blood and inflammatory cells into the urinary space (i.e., the space between Bowman's capsule and the glomerular capillary tufts). A hypercellular crescentlike, tissue appears, explaining why this form of glomerulonephritis is called crescentic. Crescentic glomerulonephritis can be also caused by other diseases, such as Wegener granulomatosis or polyarteritis nodosa, which are also diseases that damage the capillary loops of the glomeruli and allow the inflammatory exudate to accumulate in the urinary space.

7. **The answer is I.** *Focal segmental glomerulosclerosis* is the most common renal complication of intravenous drug abuse. The pathogenesis of this disease is not fully understood. Morphologically, the condition is focal and segmental (i.e., only segments of some glomeruli are hyalinized).

Clinically, it presents with proteinuria, which occasionally may be so massive as to produce nephrotic syndrome.

8. **The answer is N.** *Nodular or diffuse glomerulosclerosis* is a renal complication of long-standing diabetes mellitus that presents clinically as proteinuria. In fact, diabetic glomerulopathy is the most common cause of nephrotic syndrome in adults in the United States. Diabetes mellitus may predispose to other renal pathologic changes, such as pyelonephritis and papillary necrosis. Overall it is the most common cause of renal failure in industrialized countries.

9. **The answer is H.** *Focal necrotizing glomerulonephritis* is one of the early features of Wegener granulomatosis. The pathogenesis of this renal disease is not known, but it is thought to be immune-mediated, since most patients have antibodies to neutrophils (ANCA). Exudation of inflammatory cells through the disrupted, segmentally necrotic basement membrane leads to the formation of crescents. Clinically, the disease presents as rapidly progressive renal failure.

10. **The answer is M.** *Minimal change disease*—also known as lipoid nephrosis, nil disease, or epithelial cell disease—is a steroid-responsive form of nephrotic syndrome, most often encountered in children. The glomeruli appear normocellular, and no pathologic changes are visible by light or immunofluorescence microscopy. By electron microscopy the glomeruli show fusion of the foot processes (podocytes) of the epithelial cells.

11. **The answer is N.** Kimmelstiel-Wilson disease is the eponym for *diabetic nodular glomerulosclerosis*. Nodular widening of the mesangial areas is associated with hyalinization of arterioles, and focal hyaline changes of Bowman's capsule. The glomerular basement membranes are thickened and hyperpermeable to albumin, which leads to proteinuria.

12. **The answer is G.** *Focal proliferative glomerulonephritis* is one of several forms of lupus nephritis. In this mild form, only some glomeruli are involved, showing segmental mesangial hypercellularity. In most instances this disease can be treated with steroids, although some cases progress to diffuse proliferative glomerulonephritis.

13. **The answer is F.** *Diffuse proliferative glomerulonephritis* is a severe form of lupus nephritis, characterized by widespread involvement of glomeruli, diffuse proliferation of mesangial and endothelial cells, and even epithelial cells. Deposits of immune complexes, visible by electron microscopy or immunofluorescence microscopy, are present on both sides of the basement membrane, in the mesangial areas, and even inside the capillary loops ("hyaline thrombi"). The thickened basement membranes of the glomeruli are colloquially known as "wire loop" lesions.

14. **The answer is A.** Acute renal failure in shock is primarily caused by changes in renal hemodynamics that follow the vasoconstriction of arterioles and shunting of blood into the medulla. This prerenal failure is marked by a severe reduction in glomerular filtration pressure, and the resulting cessation of ultrafiltration through the glomeruli is reflected in *oliguria* or anuria.

15. **The answer is D.** The nephrotic syndrome is primarily marked by extensive loss of protein in the urine. Typically, the patient has *proteinuria* "in the nephrotic range," which in adults means more than 3 grams of protein in urine collected over 24 hours. Most of it is albumin, whose loss

results in hypoalbuminenmia. Disturbances in serum protein balance are accompanied by an elevation of serum cholesterol (hyperlipidemia). Edema develops owing to decreased plasma oncotic pressure.

16. **The answer is C.** *Rapidly progressive glomerulonephritis* (RPGN) is the clinical term used to denote the rapid onset of renal failure caused by severe glomerular disease. Damage to the glomeruli leads to the formation of *crescents*, and crescentic glomerulonephritis is the most common underlying cause of this clinical syndrome. Since the crescents fill the glomerular urinary space and compress the tuft, glomerular filtration is impaired. RPGN, therefore, presents with oliguria and even anuria.

17. **The answer is A.** Most ectopic kidneys are located along the pathway of renal migration during fetal development and are *caudal* to their normal lumbar position. During fetal life, the kidneys are initially located in the lower abdomen. As development progresses, they slowly move upward toward their permanent position. Kidneys that do not reach the lumbar area but remain in the pelvis or presacral area are considered ectopic.

18. **The answer is A.** *Adult polycystic kidney disease* is a mendelian autosomal dominant trait. Although the defective gene is present from birth, clinical symptoms appear only in the late twenties or thirties. The kidneys enlarge and slowly lose function; by age 40 to 50 years they have been transformed into aggregates of fluid-filled cysts. These nonfunctioning kidneys may measure 20 to 30 cm in length (normal 10 to 12 cm) and weigh up to 4500 g (normal 150 g).

19. **The answer is B.** In *systemic lupus erythematosus*, immune complexes formed against DNA, RNA, and autologous proteins may be deposited along the basement membrane of the glomeruli to form a pattern that may be indistinguishable from that of idiopathic membranous nephropathy. In contrast to other proliferative forms of lupus nephritis, mesangial cells are usually not increased in number. Unlike idiopathic membranous nephropathy, the membranous nephropathy of lupus usually displays focal mesangial deposits of immunoglobulins.

20. **The answer is C.** Acute pyelonephritis and chronic pyelonephritis are bacterial diseases that usually develop from ascending infections related to the reflux of infected urine from the lower urinary tract. *E. coli*, *Pseudomonas*, and other *Gram-negative* bacteria are the most common cause of these infections. Hematogenous dissemination of organisms is occasionally incriminated, but lymphatic spread is not thought to be important. Stagnation of urine predisposes to infection. Persistent or recurrent acute infection may lead to chronic pyelonephritis.

21. **The answer is C.** *Acute tubulointerstitial nephritis*, with dense cellular infiltrates, is typical of allergic, drug-induced, kidney disease. Eosinophils may be present but are not essential for the diagnosis of drug-induced nephropathy.

22. **The answer is D.** *Leukemic patients* who undergo chemotherapy develop hyperuricemia, owing to the increased formation of uric acid from nucleic acids released from destroyed leukemic cells. This oversupply of urates may cause renal changes similar to those of gout or other forms of hyperuricemia.

23. **The answer is D.** *Bilateral renal cortical necrosis* is a syndrome characterized by massive tubular necrosis involving large portions of the cortex

of both kidneys. Thus the difference between cortical necrosis and acute tubular necrosis is quantitative rather than qualitative. Both are most often caused by shock-related circulatory disturbances, but they also can be caused by poisoning. Massive bilateral renal cortical necrosis typically occurs in pregnancy, as a result of abruptio placentae and associated disseminated intravascular coagulation.

24. **The answer is B.** *Malignant hypertension* produces typical changes in the arterioles, which include fibrinoid necrosis and proliferation of vascular cells. This results in the so-called onion-ring hyperplastic arteriolitis. Identical findings are seen in scleroderma. By contrast, benign hypertension is associated with hyaline thickening of the arteriolar wall, and fibrinoid necrosis and cellular proliferation are not seen.

25. **The answer is A.** *Calcium oxalate* stones are the most common (80%) form of kidney stones in the United States, whereas calcium phosphate stones are more common in England. Both are usually related to idiopathic calciuria and increased absorption of calcium in the intestine. Magnesium ammonium phosphate stones are typically formed in urine made alkaline by urea-splitting bacteria. They form the so-called staghorn calculi that fill the entire pelvis and calices. Uric acid stones, found in 25% of patients with gout, are smooth, yellow, hard, and radiolucent. These stones often contain calcium, and mixed uric acid/calcium stones may be seen by x-ray. Cystine stones occur in children with hereditary cystinuria, an inborn error of amino acid metabolism marked by an excess of cystine in the urine.

26. **The answer is B.** Renal cell carcinoma originates from *renal tubules* and is composed of cuboidal cells that form either tubules or solid nests. These cells usually have a clear cytoplasm. The cytoplasm appears clear because it is rich in glycogen and fat, which are usually washed out during histologic processing of the tissue.

27. **The answer is B.** *Wilms tumor* consists histologically of immature cells similar to those in the renal primordium or immature renal tubules, glomeruli, and stroma.

28. **The answer is B.** Carcinomas of the renal pelvis present histologically as *transitional cell tumors*. Like most other urothelial tumors, they grow as papillary exophytic lesions.

Chapter 17

The Urinary Tract and Male Reproductive System

Questions

DIRECTIONS: Match each numbered statement with the most appropriate lettered item. Each lettered item can be used once, more than once, or not at all.

Renal Pelvis and Ureter

  A. Megaloureter
  B. Endometriosis
  C. Brunn nests
  D. All of the above
  E. None of the above

_____ **1.** Results from chronic inflammation
_____ **2.** Malignant
_____ **3.** Congenital
_____ **4.** Possible cause of bilateral hydronephrosis
_____ **5.** Extrinsic cause of hydronephrosis

Urinary Tract Carcinoma

  A. Carcinoma of the ureter
  B. Carcinoma of the urinary bladder
  C. Both
  D. Neither

_____ **6.** Most often transitional cell carcinoma
_____ **7.** Most often exophytic and polypoid
_____ **8.** May be accompanied by carcinoma in situ
_____ **9.** Multiple tumors commonly occur in the same patient

_____ **10.** Prognosis depends on the stage and grade of tumor
_____ **11.** Peak incidence in the early 30s
_____ **12.** Hematuria a common feature
_____ **13.** Unilateral hydroureter develops early in the disease
_____ **14.** May present as squamous carcinoma or adenocarcinoma, albeit rarely

Urinary Bladder Inflammation

    A. Acute cystitis
    B. Chronic cystitis
    C. Both
    D. Neither

_____ **15.** In the age group from 20 to 50 years, more common in women than in men
_____ **16.** Most often caused by coliform bacteria
_____ **17.** Mucosal ulcer may be associated with negative urine cultures
_____ **18.** Malakoplakia
_____ **19.** Cytotoxic drug therapy
_____ **20.** Indwelling catheter
_____ **21.** Honeymoon cystitis
_____ **22.** Tendency for recurrence or exacerbation

Testicular Lesions (Nonneoplastic)

    A. Cryptorchidism
    B. Acute orchitis
    C. Both
    D. Neither

_____ **23.** Infertility may be a consequence
_____ **24.** Increased incidence of tumors
_____ **25.** May be bilateral or unilateral
_____ **26.** Painful testis
_____ **27.** Interstitial lymphocytic infiltrates
_____ **28.** Congenital
_____ **29.** Common testicular lesion in children under 1 year of age
_____ **30.** May resolve spontaneously
_____ **31.** Surgical treatment indicated
_____ **32.** Typical feature of Klinefelter syndrome

Testicular Tumors

    A. Seminoma
    B. Teratoma

C. Embryonal carcinoma
D. Mixed germ cell tumor
E. Leydig cell tumor

_____ 33. Not a germ cell tumor
_____ 34. The most common tumor of the testis
_____ 35. The stroma of the tumor is infiltrated with lymphocytes
_____ 36. Contains intestinal, squamous, and cartilaginous tissue
_____ 37. Contains cells that secrete α-fetoprotein
_____ 38. Produces chorionic gonadotropin
_____ 39. Secretes steroid hormones
_____ 40. Causes gynecomastia

Prostatic Disease

A. Prostatic carcinoma
B. Benign prostatic hyperplasia
C. Both
D. Neither

_____ 41. Composed of cells forming glands in a fibromuscular stroma
_____ 42. Perineural infiltration
_____ 43. More common in middle age (30 to 50 years) than in old age (70 to 80 years)
_____ 44. Caused by excess androgen
_____ 45. Originates predominantly in the peripheral portions of the prostate
_____ 46. Prostate specific antigen may be elevated in serum
_____ 47. May be associated with elevation of alkaline phosphatase in serum
_____ 48. Urinary tract obstruction is an early finding
_____ 49. Secretes sex hormones
_____ 50. May be detected by rectal palpation

Answers

1. **The answer is C.** *Brunn nests* are composed of urothelium that is detached from the surface epithelium. Chronic inflammation of the renal pelvis and ureter is associated with the formation of Brunn nests.

2. **The answer is E.** *None of the lesions* listed is malignant, and even the metaplastic changes such as Brunn nests or foci of squamous epithelium are not considered premalignant.

3. **The answer is A.** *Megaloureter* is a congenital defect that can be one-sided or bilateral.

4. **The answer is A.** Increased pressure of fluid in the *dilated ureter* may cause dilatation of the renal pelvis (i.e., hydronephrosis).

5. **The answer is B.** *Endometriosis* is typically located in the periureteric space, from which it compresses the ureters externally.

6. **The answer is C.** Since the ureters and the urinary bladder are lined by *the same type* of transitional epithelium, it is not surprising that tumors in these two locations have many features in common. Thus most tumors (90%) are transitional cell carcinomas. The tumors are often multiple and may be either synchronous or metachronous (i.e., appear simultaneously or sequentially).

7. **The answer is C.** *Both tumors* are characterized by an exophytic papillary growth pattern.

8. **The answer is C.** The transitional epithelium *adjacent to the tumor* may contain carcinoma in situ. Since this lesion may not be appreciated by cystoscopy, the nonpapillomatous (i.e., flat) epithelium surrounding carcinoma of the ureter or urinary bladder should always be subjected to biopsy.

9. **The answer is C.** Urinary tract cancers are often *multifocal.*

10. **The answer is C.** The prognosis of all *transitional cell carcinomas* depends on the histologic staging and the clinical grading of the tumor.

11. **The answer is D.** Transitional carcinomas are tumors of middle-aged and older persons; *they do not occur in young adults.*

12. **The answer is C.** Hematuria is a common presenting symptom of *all* urinary tract tumors.

13. **The answer is A.** Hydroureter (i.e., dilatation of the ureter above a lesion) occurs in association with papillary *tumors of the ureter*. It is true that cancers of the urinary bladder may produce similar symptoms if located at the vesical orifice of the ureter, but this occurs rarely. Hydronephrosis occurs in late stages of bladder cancer.

14. **The answer is C.** *All malignant tumors* of the ureter and urinary bladder are squamous cell carcinomas or, even more rarely, adenocarcinomas. Squamous cell carcinomas presumably originate from foci of squamous metaplasia in chronic inflammation or in association with urolithiasis. Adenocarcinomas originate from various glandular inclusions (cystitis glandularis) and metaplastic glandlike epithelium.

15. **The answer is C.** In the age group from 20 to 50 years *all forms of cystitis* are more common in women, who have a shorter urethra and are more prone to infection than men.

16. **The answer is C.** *Both acute and chronic cystitis* are caused by the same coliform bacilli.

17. **The answer is B.** Mucosal ulcer (Hunner ulcer), usually in the dome of the bladder, occurs in middle-aged women who have no bacteriologic evidence of infection. It is a *chronic cystitis* of unknown etiology, which does not respond to chemotherapy.

18. **The answer is B.** Malakoplakia is a form of *chronic cystitis* in which the wall of the bladder is infiltrated by macrophages. These cells contain diagnostic cytoplasmic inclusions called *Michaelis-Gutmann bodies.* It is thought that the macrophages are functionally impaired and that the

cytoplasmic bodies form within their enormously enlarged lysosomes or phagosomes.

19. **The answer is B.** Cytotoxic therapy, especially with certain drugs, such as cyclophosphamide, causes *chronic cystitis* with mucosal hemorrhage, ulceration, and epithelial cytologic alterations bordering on atypia. It seems that the metabolic degradation products of the drug are excreted in urine and adversely affect the transitional epithelium of the urinary bladder.

20. **The answer is C.** Indwelling catheters can cause *both acute and chronic cystitis.*

21. **The answer is A.** "Honeymoon cystitis" is an *acute infection* after initial sexual intercourse in women who have not previously been sexually active.

22. **The answer is C.** *All urinary tract infections* have a tendency to recur.

23. **The answer is C.** *Cryptorchid testes* and those affected by various *infections* may lose germ cells, with consequent infertility.

24. **The answer is A.** There is an increased incidence of germ cell tumors in *cryptorchid testes,* but not in those afflicted by orchitis.

25. **The answer is C.** *Both cryptorchidism and orchitis* may be bilateral or unilateral. Cryptorchidism is more often unilateral. Ascending infections, such as gonorrhea and even hematogenous tuberculosis, most often cause unilateral orchitis. On the other hand, some infections, such as mumps or syphilis, generally cause bilateral orchitis.

26. **The answer is B.** *Orchitis* causes enlargement of the testis, owing to edema and inflammation. Swelling of the parenchyma distends the inelastic tunica albuginea and results in pain.

27. **The answer is B.** Lymphocytic infiltrates are found in acute mumps *orchitis* but are not seen in cryptorchidism.

28. **The answer is A.** *Cryptorchidism* is in most instances congenital. However, since the inguinal canals remain open in 3% to 4% of all male infants for at least a few months, the definitive diagnosis of cryptorchidism should be postponed until the end of the first year. Many of the retracted or inguinal testes descend into the scrotum during the first year after birth. Therefore the true incidence of cryptorchidism is only 10% of all infants who have the testis outside of the scrotum at the time of birth.

29. **The answer is A.** *Cryptorchidism* is the most common testicular lesion in children younger than 1 year.

30. **The answer is C.** *Both orchitis,* especially the viral form, and *cryptorchidism* may resolve spontaneously.

31. **The answer is A.** Acute orchitis is not treated surgically. Orchidopexy (i.e., surgical repositioning of the testis into the scrotum) is indicated for *cryptorchidism* in early childhood.

32. **The answer is D.** Although the testes in patients with Klinefelter syndrome are atrophic, they are *neither cryptorchid nor inflamed.*

33. **The answer is E.** *Leydig cell tumors* originate from the interstitial cells of the testis that produce sex hormones. Thus they are not germ cell tumors.

34. **The answer is A.** *Seminoma* is the most common testicular tumor, accounting for almost one-half of all neoplasms.

35. **The answer is A.** The stroma of *seminomas* is fibrovascular and densely infiltrated with lymphocytes, which most likely represent an immune response to the tumor.

36. **The answer is B.** *Teratomas* are composed of various somatic tissues that originate from the three primordial germinal layers: (1) intestinal-like tissue originating from endoderm, (2) squamous epithelium originating from ectoderm, and (3) cartilage originating from mesoderm. The tumors may contain other tissues and even organoid structures.

37. **The answer is D.** α-Fetoprotein is a marker of yolk sac elements, which can form a pure yolk sac tumor or be admixed with other components of a *mixed germ cell tumor.*

38. **The answer is D.** Chorionic gonadotropin is secreted by normal placental cells, choriocarcinoma, and trophoblastic components of *mixed germ cell tumors.*

39. **The answer is E.** Steroid hormones are produced by *Leydig cell tumors,* which functionally resemble normal Leydig cells of the testis.

40. **The answer is E.** Some *Leydig cell tumors* produce predominantly androgens, others synthesize a mixture of androgens and estrogens, and still others release predominantly estrogens. Excess estrogen produced by these tumors may cause feminization and gynecomastia.

41. **The answer is C.** *Both the hyperplastic* prostate and the *neoplastic* prostate contain glands. The hyperplastic glands resemble those in the normal prostate and are usually surrounded by a hyperplastic fibromuscular stroma. Similar to the normal prostate, these glands have a cuboidal inner layer surrounded by a thin outer layer composed of myoepithelial cells. By contrast, neoplastic glands are arranged as a single cell layer and are not lined by myoepithelial cells.

42. **The answer is A.** In *prostate adenocarcinoma,* the tumor cells penetrate into the surrounding tissues and commonly invade the nerves.

43. **The answer is C.** *Both prostatic hyperplasia and prostatic carcinoma* are more common in older than in younger men.

44. **The answer is D.** The cause of both of these conditions *is not known.* Although hormones play a role, it is likely that a relative decrease in androgens or an increase in estrogens causes hyperplasia. There are few clues to the cause of prostatic cancer.

45. **The answer is A.** *Prostatic carcinoma* originates predominantly in the outer portions of the prostate, whereas hyperplasia tends to involve the periurethral region.

46. **The answer is C.** Prostate specific antigen (PSA) is an organ-specific marker for prostatic disorders. High levels of PSA in the serum are typical of *prostatic carcinoma, but hyperplasia* also may cause a mild to moderate elevation.

47. **The answer is A.** Osteoblastic lesions, especially in the lumbar vertebra or the sacral bone, are typical of metastatic *prostatic carcinoma*. Metastases to bone stimulate new bone formation, which contributes to the opacification of the bone by x-ray. In the serum an increased level of alkaline phosphatase reflects release of the enzyme from osteoblasts.

48. **The answer is B.** Urinary tract obstruction is more common in patients with *benign prostatic hyperplasia* than in those with cancer, because hyperplasia predominantly involves the periurethral portion of the gland. However, advanced cancer, owing to its invasive properties and unlimited growth potential, may also produce obstruction of the urethra or invasion of the urinary bladder.

49. **The answer is D.** The prostate *does not secrete sex hormones*. Accordingly, neither benign prostatic hyperplasia nor prostate cancer secretes sex hormones.

50. **The answer is C.** Rectal palpation is the most important approach to *diagnosing prostatic disease* and is an effective means of detecting enlargement of the gland. The hyperplastic prostate is nodular and soft, whereas prostatic carcinoma presents as a focal or diffuse hardening of the gland. Since cancer originates in the peripheral portion and is often found in the "posterior lobe," rectal examination frequently provides the first evidence of this cancer.

Chapter 18

Gynecologic Pathology

Questions

DIRECTIONS: Choose the one best answer.

_____ 1. The development of which structure will be inhibited by the müllerian inhibiting substance?
A. Uterus
B. Ovary
C. Testis
D. Vulva
E. Bartholin glands

_____ 2. Which of the following epithelia is most resistant to gonorrhea?
A. Vagina in prepubertal girls
B. Vagina of sexually mature women
C. Endocervix
D. Endometrium
E. Fallopian tube

_____ 3. Which of the following infectious agents has been suggested as a cause of cervical intraepithelial neoplasia (CIN)?
A. *Mycoplasma hominis*
B. *Chlamydia trachomatis*
C. Human papilloma virus
D. *Gardnerella vaginalis*
E. *Trichomonas vaginalis*

_____ 4. All the following are typical of carcinoma of the vulva *except*
A. Peak incidence occurs in premenopausal women.
B. Squamous cell carcinoma is the most common histologic type.
C. Approximately two-thirds are exophytic.
D. Itching of long duration is a common symptom.
E. Small tumors without lymph node involvement have a good prognosis.

_____ 5. All the following apply to vaginal adenosis *except*
   A. it is a consequence of exposure to diethylstilbestrol (DES) in utero.
   B. it is more common if DES was given in early stages rather than late stages of pregnancy.
   C. the incidence correlates positively with the total amount of DES given during pregnancy.
   D. it is lined by columnar epithelium.
   E. there is a high incidence of adenocarcinoma.

_____ 6. Which of the following risk factors correlates best with the development of cervical intraepithelial neoplasia (CIN)?
   A. Coitus at early age and multiple sexual partners
   B. Cigarette smoking
   C. Gonorrhea
   D. Oral contraceptives
   E. Intravaginal contraceptives

_____ 7. All the following are true for invasive carcinoma of the cervix *except*
   A. it is more common in the United States than in Central America.
   B. peak incidence occurs at about 50 years.
   C. vaginal bleeding is the most common symptom.
   D. it originates predominantly in the transformation zone of the cervix.
   E. it usually presents as large cell nonkeratinizing carcinoma.

_____ 8. The most common cause of death in advanced cervical carcinoma is
   A. brain metastases.
   B. lung metastases.
   C. renal failure.
   D. vertebral fractures.
   E. adrenal cortical failure.

_____ 9. The best prognostic indicator of survival in patients with cervical neoplasia is
   A. exfoliative cytology findings.
   B. small cell rather than large cell carcinoma.
   C. degree of keratinization of the tumor.
   D. clinical staging of the tumor.
   E. presence of CEA (carcinoembryonic antigen) in serum.

DIRECTIONS: Match each numbered statement with the most appropriate lettered item. Each lettered item can be used once, more than once, or not at all.

Carcinoma of the Uterus

   A. Squamous cell carcinoma of the cervix
   B. Adenocarcinoma of the endometrium
   C. Both
   D. Neither

_____ 10. Related to estrogen levels
_____ 11. Can present with vaginal bleeding or spotting
_____ 12. Can be detected by exfoliative cytology
_____ 13. Preceded by intraepithelial preneoplastic lesions
_____ 14. Prognosis more dependent on staging than on histologic grading
_____ 15. Incidence increased in women on estrogen supplementation therapy

Ovarian Tumors of Surface (Germinal) Epithelium

A. Serous cystadenocarcinoma
B. Mucinous cystadenocarcinoma
C. Endometrioid adenocarcinoma
D. Clear cell adenocarcinoma
E. Brenner tumor

_____ 16. Most common malignant tumor of the ovary
_____ 17. Most common bilateral malignant tumor
_____ 18. Pseudomyxoma peritonei is a complication
_____ 19. Most common cancer that synchronously appears in the ovary and the uterus
_____ 20. Benign solid tumor

Sex Cord Stromal Tumors of the Ovary

A. Granulosa cell tumor
B. Thecoma
C. Sertoli-Leydig cell tumor
D. Fibroma
E. None of the above

_____ 21. Virilization common
_____ 22. Most efficient estrogen producer
_____ 23. Grayish-white on cross section
_____ 24. Composed of spindle-shaped, lipid-laden cells
_____ 25. Often bilateral

Germ Cell Tumors of the Ovary

A. Cystic teratoma
B. Endodermal sinus tumor (yolk sac carcinoma)
C. Choriocarcinoma
D. Dysgerminoma
E. None of the above

_____ 26. May contain skin, teeth, and cartilage
_____ 27. Most common ovarian tumor in women younger than 25 years

_____ **28.** Rarely undergoes malignant transformation
_____ **29.** Highly radiosensitive
_____ **30.** Produces α-fetoprotein
_____ **31.** Cause of a positive pregnancy test in a nonpregnant woman

Placental Disorders

A. Placenta previa
B. Placenta accreta
C. Placenta previa and placenta accreta
D. Placental infarct
E. Retroplacental hematoma

_____ **32.** Absence of decidua basalis
_____ **33.** Caused by premature placental separation
_____ **34.** Significant complication of eclampsia
_____ **35.** Cause of uterine rupture
_____ **36.** Postpartum bleeding may necessitate hysterectomy.
_____ **37.** Cause of bleeding in pregnancy

Gestational Trophoblastic Disease

A. Hydatidiform mole, complete
B. Choriocarcinoma
C. Both
D. Neither

_____ **38.** Increased serum chorionic gonadotropin
_____ **39.** Symptoms begin in the first 3 weeks of pregnancy.
_____ **40.** Tendency to metastasize
_____ **41.** Most are androgenetic in origin and homozygous.
_____ **42.** May develop after delivery

Answers

1. **The answer is A.** Müllerian inhibiting substance is produced by Sertoli cells in the testis of the male fetus. It causes involution of the Müllerian ducts, the precursors of the fallopian ducts, *uterus*, and upper third of the vagina. The formation of the ovary, testis, vulva, and Bartholin glands is not affected.

2. **The answer is B.** *Neisseria gonorrhoeae* usually invades the female genital organs through the columnar epithelium lining the endocervix, endometrium, and fallopian tubes. The squamous epithelium of the vagina of adult women keratinizes under the influence of estrogens and

is resistant to infection. However, in young girls, the epithelium is not keratinized and is susceptible to gonorrheal infection.

3. **The answer is C.** Certain types of *human papillomavirus* (16, 18, and 31) are often found in CIN and invasive carcinoma of the cervix. This virus is a known cause of venereal warts (condyloma accuminatum) and has a possible role in cervical malignancy. The other organisms listed are common causes of sexually transmitted diseases, but they have not been linked to cervical cancer.

4. **The answer is A.** Squamous cell carcinoma of the vulva occurs in women who are older than those with carcinoma of the cervix. It is a tumor of postmenopausal women, the peak incidence being *at 65 years*.

5. **The answer is E.** *Only 0.1%* of all women exposed to DES in utero develop invasive *adenocarcinoma*, whereas adenosis is found in a third of the same population. Thus malignant transformation of adenosis is rare.

6. **The answer is A.** *Early sexual activity and promiscuity* show the strongest correlation with the development of CIN. Many women who develop cervical cancer also contract sexually transmitted diseases, including the potentially carcinogenic human papillomavirus. Cigarette smoking may increase the risk of CIN somewhat, but it is not as important.

7. **The answer is A.** The incidence of carcinoma of the cervix has *decreased in the United States*, but it is still common in underdeveloped countries. Better sexual hygiene, improved screening, and early clinical detection of preinvasive lesions in the United States have contributed to the decline in incidence. In the United States, the incidence peaks at about 50 years of age (i.e., 20 years after the peak of CIN). The lesions may be exophytic or ulcerated and bleed spontaneously or during intercourse. Typically, they originate at the transformation zone of the cervix, the location of most of the reserve cells. Most cervical cancers are squamous cell carcinomas. There are three histologic types: large cell nonkeratinizing, large cell keratinizing, and small cell carcinoma.

8. **The answer is C.** Cervical cancer tends to spread by local extension and by means of pelvic lymphatics. As a result, compression of the ureters occurs frequently. The ensuing *renal failure* accounts for death in about half of all patients with cervical cancer. Distant hematogenous metastases are less common.

9. **The answer is D.** The extent of cervical cancer at the time of diagnosis (*stage*) is the best prognostic measure for the survival of the patient. Patients with stage I cancer have a 90% probability of surviving 5 years, whereas those with stage IV tumor have only a 10% chance. Histologic or cytologic findings are of secondary importance. CEA is typically not secreted by squamous carcinoma cells.

10. **The answer is B.** Estrogen is a potent proliferative stimulus for *endometrial cells* and thereby increases the incidence of malignant transformation. It has no comparable effect on the cervical epithelium.

11. **The answer is C.** *Both cervical and endometrial tumors* commonly present with bleeding.

12. **The answer is C.** *Both cervical and endometrial cancer* can be recognized by exfoliative cytology, since the cells are shed into the uterine/vaginal fluid.

13. **The answer is C.** Carcinoma of the cervix is preceded by well-defined preneoplastic lesions, known as *dysplasia* and *carcinoma in situ* or by the acronym *CIN* (cervical intraepithelial neoplasia). Complex *atypical hyperplasia* of the endometrium is a preneoplastic condition, but at times it cannot be clearly distinguished from early carcinoma.

14. **The answer is C.** Prognosis of *all gynecologic cancers* depends more on the stage than on the grade of tumors.

15. **The answer is B.** Exogenous estrogens increase the risk of *endometrial carcinoma*.

16. **The answer is A.** Serous tumors are the most common ovarian neoplasms that originate from the germinal epithelium. *Serous cystadenocarcinomas* account for 40% of all ovarian cancers.

17. **The answer is A.** Many ovarian tumors are bilateral, owing to synchronous occurrence or metastatic spread. *Serous cystadenocarcinomas* are the most common bilateral tumors, occurring in 30% of cases.

18. **The answer is B.** Pseudomyxoma peritonei is a condition characterized by mucin-rich fluid that fills the peritoneal cavity. This fluid is secreted by serosal implants of malignant tumor cells, a typical feature of peritoneal seeding of *mucinous cystadenocarcinoma*.

19. **The answer is C.** *Endometrioid carcinoma* of the ovary is histologically indistinguishable from adenocarcinoma of the endometrium. Tumors involving both the ovary and the uterus are found in 20% to 30% of patients with these neoplasms. In such instances, it is not possible to determine whether the ovarian tumor has metastasized to the uterus, or vice versa, or whether the tumors arose simultaneously.

20. **The answer is E.** *Brenner tumors* are small, solid, benign neoplasms of the ovary. They are easily distinguished microscopically from other solid malignant ovarian cancers such as endometrioid or clear cell carcinomas or metastases from other sites.

21. **The answer is C.** *Sertoli-Leydig cell tumors* typically produce androgens and cause virilization.

22. **The answer is B.** Most sex cord tumors except fibromas produce steroid hormones, but *thecomas* are most efficient in producing estrogens.

23. **The answer is D.** *Fibromas* of the ovary, like fibromas in other sites, are composed of fibroblasts surrounded by collagen and appear grayish white.

24. **The answer is B.** *Thecomas* are composed of lipid-laden spindle cells.

25. **The answer is E.** *Most sex cord stromal tumors are solitary and unilateral.*

26. **The answer is A.** Ovarian *teratomas* are benign tumors that are known as *dermoid tumors* because they almost invariably contain skin and dermal appendages. Cartilage and teeth are also common in these tumors.

27. **The answer is A.** *Teratomas* are the most common ovarian tumors in young women, accounting for 60% to 70% of all tumors in that age group.

28. **The answer is A.** *Cystic teratomas* rarely undergo malignant transformation.

29. **The answer is D.** *Dysgerminoma*, the ovarian counterpart of seminoma, is radiosensitive, a property that accounts for a good prognosis, even in large, bulky tumors.

30. **The answer is B.** α-Fetoprotein is produced in fetal life by the yolk sac and the liver. Cells resembling these fetal structures occur in some malignant germ cell tumors, most notably *endodermal sinus tumors*. Thus α-fetoprotein is a useful marker to follow patients with this tumor.

31. **The answer is C.** *Choriocarcinomas* secrete human chorionic gonadotropin and thus cause a positive pregnancy test.

32. **The answer is C.** *Placenta previa and placenta accreta* are abnormalities of placental insertion caused by the absence of decidualization at the site of implantation. Placenta previa overlies the cervix and can cause massive hemorrhage from its basal part.

33. **The answer is E.** *Retroplacental hematoma* is an important complication of premature placental separation (abruptio placentae).

34. **The answer is E.** *Retroplacental hematomas* occur more commonly in preeclampsia and eclampsia than in normal pregnancies.

35. **The answer is B.** *Placenta accreta* is characterized by the penetration of placental villi into the deeper layers of the myometrium, where they may cause uterine rupture during pregnancy.

36. **The answer is B.** Fragments of *placenta accreta* may remain after the major portion of the placenta has separated from the uterus and has been delivered with the fetus. Such residual portions of the placenta may cause postpartum hemorrhage that is difficult to control. Hysterectomy is occasionally the only way to stop the bleeding.

37. **The answer is C.** *Both placenta previa and placenta accreta* may cause bleeding in pregnancy.

38. **The answer is C.** *All forms of gestational trophoblastic disease* cause elevations of serum chorionic gonadotropin.

39. **The answer is D.** Hydatidiform mole presents as a *midgestational* enlargement of the uterus disproportional to the gestational age. Choriocarcinoma is a feature of late pregnancy or the *postpartum period*.

40. **The answer is B.** Hydatidiform moles are not malignant, whereas all *choriocarcinomas* are malignant and tend to metastasize.

41. **The answer is A.** *Hydatidiform moles* develop by androgenesis, a process akin to parthenogenetic activation of the ovum. In androgenesis, the fertilized egg loses its maternal set of chromosomes, and the paternal set undergoes reduplication. Thus the cells of a hydatidiform mole display the normal number of chromosomes (i.e., 46). In most instances, they contain two paternal X chromosomes, and the karyotype is 46,XX. The 46,YY karyotype is not viable and is aborted early. Some moles show mosaicism, or a 46,XY karyotype, which is thought to be due to fertilization of the egg with two spermatozoa, followed by the loss of maternal chromosomes.

42. **The answer is B.** *Hydatidiform mole* is a lesion of pregnancy and does not develop postpartum. On the other hand, 50% of choriocarcinomas develop after delivery of a normal baby or after an abortion. The remaining half develop from preceding hydatiform moles.

The Breast

Questions

Tumors and Tumorlike Lesions of the Breast

A. Colloid carcinoma
B. Fibroadenoma
C. Fibrocystic change
D. Intraductal carcinoma
E. Intraductal papilloma
F. Invasive ductal carcinoma
G. Invasive lobular carcinoma
H. Lobular carcinoma in situ
I. Medullary carcinoma
J. Paget disease
K. Phyllodes tumor
L. Tubular carcinoma

_____ 1. A 35-year-old nulliparous woman complained that her breasts were swollen and nodular upon palpation. A mammogram disclosed foci of calcification, and a biopsy showed fibrosis, dilatation of ducts, foci of apocrine metaplasia, and areas of sclerosing adenosis.

_____ 2. A 5-cm, well-encapsulated nodule was removed from the breast of a 25-year-old woman. Histologically, the mass was composed of elongated, ductlike structures surrounded by loose fibrous connective tissue.

_____ 3. A 55-year-old woman complained of bloody discharge from her left nipple. A 1-cm nodule was removed from the subareolar breast tissue. Histologically, the tumor was composed of cuboidal and myoepithelial cells that lined vascular connective tissue cores and projected into the lumen of a major lactiferous duct.

_____ 4. A 45-year-old woman had an area of calcification in her left breast demonstrated by mammography. A breast biopsy disclosed that the ducts contained anastomosing strands of neoplastic cells, forming a cribriform pattern. The tumor contained foci of necrosis, but there was no evidence of invasive growth.

_____ 5. A biopsy was performed to remove a 2-cm, rock-hard mass from the breast of a 50-year-old woman. The tumor was composed of cuboidal cells that formed ductlike or glandlike structures and solid nests surrounded by dense collagenous stroma.

_____ 6. A biopsy performed on a 52-year-old woman revealed that her breast was infiltrated with small cuboidal cells, with round nuclei and prominent nucleoli, which were arranged in single cell columns between strands of connective tissue. The adjacent lobules were filled with compact groups of similar cells.

_____ 7. A 5-cm soft mass was removed from the breast of a 50-year-old woman. Histologically, the tumor was composed of clusters of vacuolated cuboidal cells floating in pools of mucus.

_____ 8. A 3-cm soft mass was removed from the breast of a 55-year-old woman. Histologically, it was composed of solid nests and sheets of neoplastic cells infiltrated at their periphery with lymphocytes.

_____ 9. A 45-year-old woman noticed an oozing reddish patch on her right nipple, which she thought was an allergic reaction to her bra. Cytologic examination of the fluid revealed malignant cells. A mastectomy specimen showed malignant cells in the lactiferous ducts, which infiltrated the epidermis of the areola.

_____ 10. A 30-year-old woman developed a large breast tumor measuring 15 cm in diameter. The mass was lobulated and was composed histologically of moderately cellular, loose connective tissue, with nodules and ridges lined by cuboidal cells.

_____ 11. A tumor measuring 3 cm in diameter was removed from the breast of a 60-year-old woman. The pathologist described the cross section as firm, gritty, and chalky white. Histologically, it displayed glandlike elements and a strong desmoplastic reaction.

DIRECTIONS: Choose the one best answer.

_____ 12. The lowest incidence of breast cancer is found in women who
A. were pregnant at an early age.
B. had early menarche.
C. had late menopause.
D. were nulliparous.
E. had carcinoma of the ovary or endometrium.

_____ 13. What proportion of American women are expected to develop breast cancer by the age of 70 years?
A. 7%
B. 15%
C. 30%
D. 50%
E. 75%

_____ **14.** Which oncogene plays a pathogenetic role in familial breast cancer?
   A. *Myc*
   B. *BRCA-1*
   C. *Ki-ras*
   D. *Abl*
   E. *Fos*

_____ **15.** Longer disease-free survival and overall survival are expected in women whose breast cancers show a high degree or level of
   A. histologic grade.
   B. nuclear atypia.
   C. estrogen receptors.
   D. EGF receptors.
   E. Her2/neu.

_____ **16.** Which of the following histologic patterns of breast carcinoma is associated with the best prognosis?
   A. Invasive ductal
   B. Invasive lobular
   C. Invasive tubular
   D. Medullary
   E. Mucinous

_____ **17.** Which of the following statements is true for breast cancer in men?
   A. It is only 1% as common as breast cancer in women.
   B. Lobular carcinoma is the most common histologic type.
   C. It is often bilateral.
   D. It has a better prognosis than breast cancer in women.
   E. It is often preceded by atypical epithelial hyperplasia.

_____ **18.** All the following are associated with a poor prognosis for breast cancer *except*
   A. a primary tumor 6 cm in diameter.
   B. cytologic anaplasia, high mitotic index, and pleomorphism.
   C. a lack of circumscription.
   D. invasion of dermal lymphatics.
   E. intraductal carcinoma.

_____ **19.** The overall 5-year survival rate for treated breast cancer in Stage I is
   A. 85%.
   B. 50%.
   C. 35%.
   D. 20%.
   E. less than 5%.

_____ **24.** Estrogen receptors are more common in
   A. breast tumors of younger rather than older women.
   B. histologically well-differentiated tumors.
   C. tumors that show DNA aneuploidy.
   D. tumors that do not respond to anti-estrogen therapy.
   E. tumors that have metastases in the liver.

Answers

1. **The answer is C.** *Fibrocystic change* of the breast, at least in the common form, involves both breasts and is dominated by fibrosis and ductal cyst formation. It is not considered to be a premalignant change. Epithelial changes such as sclerosing adenosis are also benign. A small minority of cases of fibrocystic change show more ominous epithelial hyperplasia, which is potentially premalignant. Epithelial hyperplasia may transform into atypical ductal and lobular hyperplasia and eventually evolve into cancer.

2. **The answer is B.** *Fibroadenomas* usually present as solitary, well-circumscribed nodules, showing proliferation of epithelial and connective-tissue elements. The peak incidence of fibroadenomas is between 20 and 35 years of age. Surgical removal is curative.

3. **The answer is E.** *Intraductual papilloma* is a benign breast tumor that usually causes nipple discharge, which may be serous or hemorrhagic.

4. **The answer is D.** *Intraductal carcinoma* grows in a cribriform pattern or may show central necrosis ("comedocarcinoma") of intraductal cell masses.

5. **The answer is F.** *Invasive ductal carcinoma* is the most common form of breast cancer and presents as a scirrhous carcinoma (i.e., it elicits a strong desmoplastic reaction). This connective-tissue response accounts for the firm consistency and color of the tumor and for the retraction of the nipple and skin overlying the tumor. Since duct carcinoma often contains microcalcifications, it may be gritty when sectioned.

6. **The answer is G.** *Lobular carcinoma* in situ originates in the lobules, whereas most breast tumors arise in the ducts. Lobular carcinoma in situ has a tendency to be bilateral and multicentric and has a better prognosis than infiltrating lobular carcinoma.

7. **The answer is A.** *Mucinous carcinoma* is a gelatinous tumor that occurs almost exclusively in older women. It has a better prognosis than infiltrating duct carcinoma.

8. **The answer is I.** *Medullary carcinomas* present as fleshy, bulky tumors measuring 5 to 10 cm in diameter. They are generally larger at the time they are detected than infiltrating duct carcinomas (average size 2–3 cm). Nevertheless, they have a somewhat better prognosis.

9. **The answer is J.** Breast cancer that involves the nipple and causes an eczema-like lesion is known as *Paget disease*. In this variant of infiltrating duct carcinoma, the cells invade the skin of the nipple. Thus its prognosis is similar to that of infiltrating duct carcinoma.

10. **The answer is K.** *Phyllodes tumor*, or giant fibroadenoma, may became large rapidly. Similar to fibroadenoma, it is composed of ductlike epithelial and stromal fibroblastic cells.

11. **The answer is F.** *Invasive ductal carcinoma* evokes a desmoplastic reaction and is therefore "rock-hard" and gritty. It is also called scirrhous carcinoma.

12. **The answer is A.** Women who are *impregnated at an early age* are at a lower risk for breast cancer than those who become pregnant later in life

or remain nulliparous. Early menarche and late menopause are associated with an increased risk of breast cancer. Carcinoma of the ovary or endometrium is also a risk factor for breast cancer.

13. **The answer is A.** Some 7% of all American women are expected to develop breast cancer by the age of 70 years.

14. **The answer is B.** *BRCA-1* and *BRCA-2* are oncogenes implicated in the pathogenesis of familial breast cancers.

15. **The answer is C.** High levels of *estrogen receptors* correlate with longer survival of breast cancer patients treated with hormnes.

16. **The answer is C.** *Tubular carcinoma* of the breast has an excellent prognosis, but it is a rare form of cancer.

17. **The answer is A.** Breast cancer in men accounts for 1% of all breast cancers. In the vast majority of cases, the tumor is an infiltrating duct carcinoma. Lobular carcinoma does not develop in the male breast. Precursor lesions, such as atypical epithelial hyperplasia of the female breast, have not been identified in men. Male tumors are typically unilateral and infiltrate rapidly into the chest muscle. The diagnosis is often delayed because of a lack of awareness of this form of cancer in men. The prognosis is actually less favorable than that for female breast cancer.

18. **The answer is E.** The first four items listed are associated with a poor prognosis. However, if the tumor is still *intraductal*, it has a good prognosis. It is important to recognize that every intraductal carcinoma should be carefully examined for possible microscopic invasion, a feature that may lead to metastasis.

19. **The answer is A.** The prognosis for breast cancer depends on the size of tumor and the presence of lymph node metastases at the time of diagnosis. Stage I tumors (i.e., those measuring less than 2 cm in diameter, without lymph node metastases) have a favorable prognosis (85% or more for 5-year survival). Early detection of breast cancer is therefore of paramount importance for successful surgical treatment.

20. **The answer is B.** Estrogen and progesterone receptors are common in *well-differentiated breast cancers of older women*. Such receptors are less frequent in tumors of premenopausal women, in anaplastic tumors that have prominent nuclear pleomorphism (reflected in chromosomal aneuploidy), and in those that have metastasized widely. Anti-estrogen therapy is effective only in tumors that express these hormone receptors.

Chapter 20

Blood and the Lymphoid Organs

DIRECTIONS: Match each numbered statement with the most appropriate lettered item. Each lettered item can be used once, more than once, or not at all.

Disorders of Red Blood Cells

A. Anemia of chronic disease
B. Anemia of chronic renal failure
C. Aplastic anemia
D. Hereditary spherocytosis
E. Glucose-6-phosphate dehydrogenase deficiency
F. Iron deficiency anemia
G. Immunohemolytic anemia, warm antibody type
H. Immunohemolytic anemia, cold agglutin type
I. Megaloblastic anemia
J. Microangiopathic hemolytic anemia
K. Myelophthisic anemia
L. Paroxysmal cold hemoglobinuria
M. Paroxysmal nocturnal hemoglobinuria
N. Polycythemia vera
O. Polycythemia, secondary
P. Sickle cell anemia
Q. Thalassemia major (Cooley anemia)
R. Thalassemia minor

_____ **1.** A 43-year-old woman of Scandinavian descent complained of constant tiredness, light-headedness, and occasional palpitations and shortness of breath while ascending the stairs. Physical examination revealed some pallor of the mucosa and a raspberry red tongue. Examination of the blood revealed a macrocytic anemia. The red blood cells showed poikilocytosis, often lacking the central pale area. Neutrophils were often hypersegmented. Serum cobalamine was low, and atrophic gastritis was diagnosed by gastric biopsy.

_____ 2. A 30-year-old woman of Vietnamese extraction complained of easy fatigability, bruising, and recurrent throat infections. Physical examination revealed numerous petechiae over her body and mouth. Abnormal laboratory findings included the following: red blood cells $3.5 \times 10^6/\mu l$; hemoglobin, 6 g/dl; white blood cells $1.5 \times 10^3/\mu l$; platelets $20 \times 10^3/\mu l$. The bone marrow biopsy revealed that hemopoietic cells had been replaced by adipocytes.

_____ 3. A 20-year-old woman complained that she could not concentrate and was always tired. She had heavy menstrual bleeding every month but was otherwise healthy. Examination of the blood showed a microcytic hypochromic anemia. A peripheral blood smear showed anisocytosis, ovalocytosis, and elliptocytosis ("pencil or cigar" cells) of red blood cells.

_____ 4. A 10-year-old boy was hospitalized for evaluation of jaundice, anemia, and splenomegaly. Laboratory studies disclosed hyperbilirubinemia and microcytic anemia. In the peripheral smear, most erythrocytes appeared round and lacked central pallor. The osmotic fragility of red blood cells was increased but the Coombs test was negative.

_____ 5. Microcytic, hypochromic anemia and jaundice were diagnosed in a 10-month-old boy of Arabic extraction who failed to thrive. Laboratory findings included red blood cell count of $2.5 \times 10^6/\mu l$. A peripheral blood smear showed marked anisopoikilocytosis, hypochromia, basophilic stippling, prominent target cells, and numerous nucleated red blood cells. A bone marrow aspirate demonstrated marked erythroid hyperplasia and increased iron stores. Electrophoresis disclosed increased amounts of fetal hemoglobin and absence of HbA.

Disorders of White Blood Cells

A. Hodgkin's disease
B. Langerhans cell histiocytosis
C. Leukemia, acute lymphoblastic
D. Leukemia, acute myelogenous
E. Leukemia, chronic lymphocytic
F. Leukemia, chronic myelogenous
G. Leukemia, hairy cell
H. Lymphadenitis
I. Lymphoma, intermediate grade
J. Lymphoma, low grade
K. Lymphoma, high grade
L. Monoclonal gammopathy of unknown significance (MGUS)
M. Multiple myeloma
N. Mycosis fungoides
O. Myelodysplastic syndrome
P. Myelofibrosis
Q. Systemic mastocytosis
R. Waldenström macroglobulinemia

_____ 6. A 60-year-old man complained of night sweats, weight loss, easy fatigability, and discomfort in the left upper abdominal quadrant. Splenomegaly was found on physical examination. Leukocytosis of $40 \times 10^3/\mu l$ was found. A peripheral blood smear showed mature and maturing granulocytes, myelocytes, basophils, and occasional myeloblasts. The bone marrow was hypercellular and dominated by white blood cell precursors. Myeloblasts and promyelocytes accounted for less than 10% of all cells. Megakaryocytes were numerous, and red blood cell precursors seemed to be less prominent. Karyotyping disclosed a monoclonal population of abnormal cells that had t(9,22) (q34; q11).

_____ 7. A 28-year-old woman felt tired and nauseated and had noticed gingival bleeding. Physical examination revealed numerous pustules on the face, splenomegaly and hepatomegaly. Laboratory findings included red blood cells $4 \times 10^6/\mu l$ and platelets $50 \times 10^3/\mu l$. A peripheral blood smear disclosed that 80% of all white blood cells were myeloblasts, 5% of which contained Auer bodies. The bone marrow contained 50% blasts, and red blood cell precursors and megakaryocytes were decreased.

_____ 8. A 60-year-old man noticed lymph node enlargement in his neck and axillae. A peripheral blood smear disclosed mild anemia and a leukocytosis of $20 \times 10^3/\mu l$. More than 80% of all white blood cells were small lymphocytes, but there were also prominent "smudge cells." The Coombs test was positive. A bone marrow biopsy contained nodular and interstitial infiltrates of lymphocytes, which showed clonal rearrangement of the IgG light-chain gene.

_____ 9. A 20-year-old woman presented with cervical adenopathy of 2 months duration. Laboratory findings were within the normal range. A lymph node biopsy showed broad bands of dense collagen subdividing the lymph node, which was infiltrated by numerous mononuclear lacunar cells and large, atypical, binucleated cells.

_____ 10. A 55-year-old man complained of pain in his back. X-ray examination revealed numerous lytic lesions in the lumbar vertebral bodies. Laboratory studies disclosed mild anemia. A monoclonal IgG spike was discovered by electrophoresis. A bone marrow biopsy disclosed foci of plasma cells, which accounted for 18% of all hematopoietic cells. The urine contained Bence Jones protein.

Bleeding Disorders

A. Antiphospholipid antibody syndrome
B. Bernard-Soulier syndrome
C. Disseminated intravascular coagulation
D. Drug-induced thrombocytopenia
E. Hemolytic uremic syndrome
F. Hemophilia A
G. Hemophilia B
H. Henoch-Schönlein purpura

    I.   Hereditary hemorrhagic telangiectasia
    J.   Idiopathic thrombocytopenic purpura, acute
    K. Idiopathic thrombocytopenic purpura, chronic
    L.   Thrombotic thrombocytopenic purpura
    M. von Willebrand disease

_____ **11.** A 9-year-old child had a bout of "flu" and suddenly developed widespread pinpoint skin hemorrhages. Laboratory findings revealed a platelet count of $20 \times 10^3/\mu l$ and no other abnormalities. The bone marrow showed an increased number of megakarocytes, which appeared mononuclear and had smooth cytoplasmic contours. The symptoms disappeared spontaneously.

_____ **12.** A 7-year-old girl was brought to the physician because her mother noticed that she bruised easily and often bled from her nose and gums. Her father and one of her four brothers had similar problems. Laboratory tests showed a prolonged bleeding time, which was even more prolonged by aspirin; prolonged partial thromboplastin time; decreased factor VIII antigen. The ristocetin cofactor assay, which measures the aggregation of fixed or washed platelets, was abnormal. The platelet count was normal. She responded well to treatment with fresh-frozen plasma.

_____ **13.** A 25-year-old woman experienced a bout of seizures, after which she was partially paralyzed but recovered. The next day she developed a fever and widespread purpura. Laboratory findings included anemia and thrombocytopenia. A peripheral blood smear contained numerous schistocytes, helmet cells, and red blood cell fragments. The blood bilirubin was elevated, and haptoglobin was undetectable. LDH, BUN, and creatinine were elevated. Coagulation tests were normal.

_____ **14.** A 4-year-old boy developed massive bleeding into the knee joint. The bleeding time, prothrombin time (PT), and platelet counts were normal, but the partial thromboplastin time (PTT) was prolonged. The blood level of factor IX was reduced, but factor VIII was normal. Mixing of the patient's blood with the blood of a control normalized the PTT.

DIRECTIONS: Choose the one best answer.

_____ **15.** In the normal hematopoietic bone marrow approximately one-half of all cells are
    A. myeloid cells.
    B. erythroid cells.
    C. megakaryocytes.
    D. plasma cells.
    E. fat cells.

_____ **16.** An increased number of reticulocytes is found in patients who have
   A. aplastic anemia.
   B. hemolytic anemia.
   C. iron deficiency anemia.
   D. anemia of chronic renal disease.
   E. myelophthisic anemia.

_____ **17.** Terminal deoxynucleotidyl transferase (Tdt) is a marker for
   A. plasma cells.
   B. neutrophils.
   C. mature T cells.
   D. mature B cells.
   E. immature pre-B and pre-T-lymphocytes.

_____ **18.** In acute or chronic idiopathic thrombocytopenic purpura, platelets are destroyed mostly in the
   A. spleen.
   B. liver.
   C. lymph nodes.
   D. bone marrow.
   E. lungs.

_____ **19.** Anemia of chronic renal failure may be caused by all the following *except*
   A. decreased erythropoietin production.
   B. bone marrow suppression by unexcreted metabolites.
   C. reduced life span of red blood cells.
   D. deficiency of iron and folic acid.
   E. immune-mediated hemolysis.

_____ **20.** Impaired production of hemoglobin A or A_2, or fetal hemoglobin, is typically found in
   A. α-thalassemia.
   B. β-thalassemia.
   C. sickle cell anemia.
   D. hereditary spherocytosis.
   E. hereditary elliptocytosis.

_____ **21.** Hereditary spherocytosis is accompanied by an increased incidence of
   A. hyperthyroidism.
   B. hypothyroidism.
   C. cholelithiasis.
   D. urinary stones.
   E. calcific aortic stenosis.

_____ **22.** Which renal disease is a complication of sickling of erythrocytes in sickle cell anemia?
   A. Acute glomerulonephritis
   B. Chronic glomerulonephritis
   C. Tubulointerstitial crystal deposition
   D. Papillary necrosis
   E. Urolithiasis

_____ 23. Most autoimmune hemolytic anemias are mediated by autoantibodies that are classified as
A. warm IgG.
B. cold IgG.
C. warm IgM.
D. cold IgM.
E. IgA.

_____ 24. Which is the most common tumor associated with secondary hemolytic anemia?
A. Carcinoma
B. Lymphoma
C. Glioma
D. Teratoma
E. Sarcoma

_____ 25. Headaches and visual problems are common symptoms of
A. aplastic anemia.
B. hemolytic anemia.
C. agranulocytosis.
D. lymphopenia.
E. polycythemia.

_____ 26. The most common cause of death in acute myelogenous leukemia (AML) is
A. bleeding.
B. thrombosis.
C. infection.
D. alkalosis.
E. acidosis.

_____ 27. The typical patient with untreated lymphocytic leukemia will die within which period after diagnosis?
A. 3–6 months
B. 6–12 months
C. 1–2 years
D. 2–3 years
E. 6–10 years

_____ 28. In hairy cell leukemia, the neoplastic cells are classified as
A. pre-B, pre-T-lymphocytes.
B. B cells.
C. T cells.
D. plasma cells.
E. myeloid precursors.

_____ 29. Cells in chronic lymphocytic leukemia are equivalent to cells of
A. Sézary syndrome.
B. mycosis fungoides.
C. small cell lymphocytic lymphoma.
D. immunoblastic lymphoma.
E. Burkitt lymphoma.

_____ **30.** The most common and ultimately lethal extramedullary complication of multiple myeloma is
A. amyloidosis of the brain.
B. amyloidosis of the liver.
C. kidney disease.
D. peritonitis.
E. pericarditis.

A n s w e r s

1. **The answer is I.** *Megaloblastic anemia* is caused by impaired DNA synthesis owing to a deficiency of vitamin B_{12} or folic acid. The peripheral blood shows macrocytosis and hypersegmentation of neutrophils. Macrocytosis accounts for the increased mean corpuscular volume. The bone marrow is hypercellular and contains megaloblasts. Vitamin B_{12} deficiency is typically caused by atrophic gastritis, which reduces the secretion of intrinsic factor and thus the absorption of vitamin B_{12}.

2. **The answer is C.** *Aplastic anemia* is a pancytopenia that results from the cessation of hemopoiesis. It probably reflects a failure of stem cells to populate the marrow. Although toxins, radiation, and viral infections can precipitate the condition, in most cases the cause of aplastic anemia is unknown. Symptoms are related to anemia, leukopenia, and thrombocytopenia.

3. **The answer is F.** *Iron deficiency anemia* is a microcytic, hypochromic anemia caused by inadequate uptake or, more often, excessive loss of iron. Women who have menorrhagia are especially prone to iron deficiency anemia. Symptoms are usually mild and nonspecific but are occasionally severe. Iron stores of the body are reduced, as evidenced by reduced levels of serum ferritin. The total iron-binding capacity of the plasma (TIBC) is usually increased, and the saturation (iron/TIBC) is low (less than 15%). The bone marrow contains decreased amounts of hemosiderin.

4. **The answer is D.** *Hereditary spherocytosis* refers to a group of hereditary hemolytic anemias caused by defects in the cytoskeleton of red blood cells. The erythrocytes are spherical and show increased osmotic fragility. Abnormal red cells are destroyed in the spleen, leading to hepatosplenomegaly and hyperbilirubinemia.

5. **The answer is Q.** *Thalassemia major* (homozygous β-thalassemia, Cooley anemia) is caused by a defect in the gene encoding the synthesis of the β chain of hemoglobin. Accordingly, hemoglobin A ($\alpha_2 \beta_2$) is not formed. Unpaired α chains precipitate in red blood cells, accounting for ineffective erythropoiesis and increased hemolysis. The red cells are hypochromic, vary in size and shape (anisocytosis and poikilocytosis), and often have a target cell configuration. Symptoms of the disease appear early in life, and affected children require constant transfusions.

6. **The answer is F.** *Chronic myelogenous leukemia* is a neoplastic disorder of multipotential hemopoietic stem cells, which show granulocytic differentiation. The bone marrow of these patients is occupied by neoplastic cells. In 90% of cases the leukemic cells contain the Philadelphia (Ph_1)

chromosome, a restructured chromosome 22 portion that has undergone reciprocal translocation with chromosome 9. The disease affects middle-aged or older adults. The initial symptoms are nonspecific and include weakness, malaise, fever, and splenomegaly. Replacement of the bone marrow by neoplastic cells causes anemia and thrombocytopenia and a predisposition to infections.

7. **The answer is D.** *Acute myelogenous leukemia* (AML) is a neoplastic disorder of the multipotential hematopoietic stem cells, which shows little or no capacity for differentiation along granulocytic, erythroid, or megakaryocytic lineages. The diagnosis is established on the basis of the peripheral smear and bone marrow biopsy, which contain blasts.

8. **The answer is E.** *Chronic lymphocytic leukemia* is characterized by clonal proliferation of small, mature-appearing lymphocytes in the bone marrow, lymph nodes, and spleen, with an expression in the peripheral blood. In most instances the leukemic cells belong to B-cell lineage and show clonal Ig gene rearrangements and activation of the *bcl* protooncogene. The disease affects men more often than women (2:1). Most patients are over 50 years. The symptoms tend to be nonspecific, but 80% of patients have lymph node enlargement and 50% show splenomegaly.

9. **The answer is A.** *Hodgkin's disease* is a lymphoid neoplasia of unknown histogenesis that is characterized by the appearance of diagnostic Reed-Sternberg cells in lymph nodes. Four histologic subtypes are recognized: lymphocyte predominant, mixed cellularity, lymphocyte depleted, and nodular sclerosis. The disease has two peaks of incidence at the ages of 20 and 60 years.

10. **The answer is M.** *Multiple myeloma* is a neoplasm of plasma cells or their B-cell precursors. Infiltrates of neoplastic plasma cells in the bone marrow cause lytic lesions, usually in the vertebrae, ribs or calvaria. A monoclonal Ig peak can be demonstrated by serum electrophoresis. IgG light chains of IgG appears in the urine of 75% of patients as Bence Jones protein.

11. **The answer is J.** *Acute idiopathic thrombocytopenic purpura* is a childhood disease that usually appears after a viral infection. Thrombocytopenia (usually $20 \times 10^3/\mu l$) is immune-mediated and accompanied by petechial hemorrhages. The bone marrow shows a compensatory hyperplasia of megakaryocytes, which appear immature. The disease tends to heal spontaneously.

12. **The answer is M.** *von Willebrand disease* is the most common hereditary bleeding disorder. It is caused by a deficiency or abnormality of von Willebrand factor (vWF), the gene for which is located on chromosome 12. Accordingly, the disease affects both males and females. Type I and II are inherited as an autosomal dominant trait, whereas type III is autosomal recessive with variable penetrance. Abnormalities of vWF affect the functions of platelets; the bleeding time and platelet aggregation induced by ristocetin are prolonged. The plasma concentration of factor VIII is reduced because vWF is a major carrier for factor VIII. Reduced levels of factor VIII below 25% of normal result in a prolonged partial thromboplastin time (PTT).

13. **The answer is L.** *Thrombotic thrombocytopenic purpura (TTP)* occurs in acute or chronic form and presents with a pentad that includes fever,

thrombocytopenia, microangiopathic hemolytic anemia, renal impairment, and neurologic symptoms. Microangiopathic hemolytic anemia presents with anemia, bilirubinemia, high LDH, reduced haptoglobin levels, and deformed red blood cells or red blood cell fragments in peripheral blood smears. Renal failure causes elevation of BUN and creatinine. TTP resembles hemolytic uremic syndrome (HUS), which occurs more often in children than in adults. HUS is often precipitated by diarrheal diseases (*E. coli*, *Salmonella typhi*, viruses) and has a good prognosis. Renal failure dominates in HUS, and there are no neurologic abnormalities.

14. **The answer is G.** *Hemophilia B* is an X-linked recessive disease caused by mutations in the gene encoding factor IX. It accounts for only 10% of all cases of hemophilia. One-third of all cases represent new mutations. It is clinically indistinguishable from hemophilia A (factor VIII deficiency). In both forms of hemophilia, the PTT is prolonged. Mixing of a patient's blood with that of a normal donor usually normalizes the PTT.

15. **The answer is E.** In the normal hemopoietic bone marrow, about one-half of all the cells are *fat cells*. There are considerably more myeloid (M) than erythroid (E) cells, and the normal M:E ratio is 2:1 to 4:1.

16. **The answer is B.** Reticulocytes are immature red blood cells. They have cytoplasmic mitochondria and ribosomes, which are eliminated during the first 1 to 2 days in the circulation. Normal peripheral blood contains less than 0.1% reticulocytes. An increased number of reticulocytes is found under conditions that promote erythropoiesis and an increased discharge of immature red blood cells from the bone marrow (e.g., *hemolytic anemia*).

17. **The answer is E.** Tdt is not found on mature lymphocytes, but rather on stem cells and *pre-B and pre-T-lymphocytes.* It is a marker that separates immature lymphoid cells and their corresponding lymphomas leukemias from immature or malignant myeloid cells, which do not express this enzyme.

18. **The answer is A.** Platelets are destroyed principally in the *spleen.* In acute idiopathic thrombocytopenic purpura (ITP) the destruction of platelets sequestered in the spleen is most likely immunologically mediated. Chronic ITP affects middle-aged women, without any preceding acute illness, and is marked by relapses and remissions. The destruction of platelets also occurs mostly in the spleen. Chronic ITP may precede a malignant lymphoma or an autoimmune disease.

19. **The answer is E.** The *anemia of chronic renal failure* has many causes, including (a) decreased production of erythropoietin by the damaged kidneys, (b) suppression of the bone marrow by residual toxic metabolites not excreted by the kidneys, (c) increased hemolysis and reduced lifespan of erythrocytes, and (d) deficiencies of iron and folic acid in patients on chronic dialysis.

20. **The answer is A.** *α-Thalassemia* is caused by deficient formation of the a-chain of hemoglobin. There is impaired production of hemoglobin A_2 ($α_2β_2$), A_2 ($α_2δ_2$), or fetal hemoglobin ($α_2γ_2$). On the other hand, since there are four genes for the α-chain, the defect may involve only one, two, or three genes and thereby cause a dose-related deficiency. Accordingly, the anemia is mild to severe. If only one α-gene is defective or missing, the patient is virtually asymptomatic; if two are mutated or

missing, there is a mild hemolytic anemia; if three are mutated or missing, excess (γ-globins form homotetramers (hemoglobin H), resulting in moderate hemolytic anemia, hypochromia, and microcytosis.

21. **The answer is C.** *Spherocytosis*, like all chronic hemolytic anemias, is associated with hyperbilirubinemia. Owing to the increased supply of bilirubin, there is an increased incidence of pigment gallstones.

22. **The answer is D.** Sickling occurs preferentially in conditions of low oxygen, low blood pH (acid), and high osmolality. Such circumstances typically occur in the renal medulla, and thus *papillary necrosis* is a complication of sickle cell anemia.

23. **The answer is A.** Most of the autoimmune hemolytic anemias are mediated by *warm IgG autoantibodies* (i.e., antibodies that exert their maximal effect at body temperature). Cold antibodies of the IgM type, which act optimally below 31°C, are less common, causing about 15% of all autoimmune hemolytic anemias.

24. **The answer is B.** The *lymphocytic lymphomas* and chronic lymphocytic leukemia account for half of all *secondary* hemolytic anemias. The remaining secondary autoimmune hemolytic anemias occur in association with other autoimmune disorders, such as systemic lupus erythematosus, viral infections, or chronic diseases of unknown origin, such as ulcerative colitis.

25. **The answer is E.** *Headaches and visual problems in polycythemia vera* are due to increased viscosity of the blood, which impedes the circulation through small blood vessels, especially those in the eye and brain.

26. **The answer is C.** The most common cause of death in acute myelogenous leukemia is *infection*, owing to a deficiency of mature granulocytes.

27. **The answer is E.** *Chronic lymphocytic leukemia* usually has an indolent and protracted course. Since the cells are well-differentiated lymphocytes, they do not respond well to chemotherapy. Thus treatment is not provided until the disease becomes incapacitating or transforms into a more aggressive, rapidly proliferating form.

28. **The answer is B.** Hairy cell leukemia in most instances is a *B-cell lymphoma*. The male-to-female ratio is 4:1, and the median age at diagnosis is 50 years. Splenomegaly is found in 85% of cases and may be massive.

29. **The answer is C.** *Diffuse small cell lymphocytic lymphoma* is composed of morphologically mature lymphocytes, corresponding to the cells of chronic lymphocytic leukemia. Similar to the latter disease, it has a good prognosis, and prolonged survival is to be expected.

30. **The answer is C.** The most common and important extramedullary complication of multiple myeloma is *kidney disease* ("myeloma kidney"), which accounts for more than half of all deaths. Other complications include bone fractures and infection. Amyloidosis occurs in various organs in 10% to 15% of cases, but it is not restricted to the brain or liver.

Chapter 21

Endocrine System

Questions

DIRECTIONS: Match each numbered statement with the most appropriate lettered item. Each lettered item can be used once, more than once, or not at all.

A. Acromegaly
B. Addison disease
C. Adrenogenital syndrome
D. Amenorrhea-galactorrhea syndrome
E. Cushing disease
F. Cushing syndrome
G. Diabetes insipidus
H. Goiter, multinodular
I. Hyperparathyroidism, primary
J. Hyperparathyroidism, secondary
K. Hyperthyroidism
L. Hypoparathyroidism
M. Hypothyroidism
N. Multiple endocrine neoplasia, type 1 (MEN-1)
O. Multiple endocrine neoplasia, type 2 (MEN-2)
P. Neuroblastoma
Q. Pheochromocytoma
R. Sheehan syndrome
S. Syndrome of inappropriate ADH secretion

_____ 1. Massive water retention in a 60-year-old man with small cell carcinoma of the lung. The patient did not have features of Cushing syndrome, and the corticosteroid levels were normal.

_____ 2. Postpartum necrosis of the pituitary

_____ 3. Paroxysmal hypertension with increased urinary catecholamines in a 50-year-old man

_____ 4. Polyuria in a man who had a trauma of the base of the skull

_____ 5. Cretinism

_____ 6. A malignant, retroperitoneal, abdominal tumor in a 4-year-old child. The tumor was composed of "small blue cells," and the urine contained increased amounts of vanillylmandelic acid.

_____ 7. An abdominal tumor originated from the para-aortic sympathetic ganglia in a 60-year-old man. By light microscopy it was composed of polygonal "chromaffin" cells, and membrane-bound granules were visible by electron microscopy. Clinically he suffered from epistatic hypertension.

_____ 8. Autoimmune adrenalitis

_____ 9. DiGeorge syndrome

_____ 10. The most common lesion of the thyroid causing a mass in the neck of middle-aged women

_____ 11. Buffalo hump, diabetes mellitus, and abdominal striae in a 40-year-old woman. Clinical workup revealed retroperitoneal abdominal tumor, which was yellow on cross section.

_____ 12. Hypercalcemia associated with a neck tumor

_____ 13. Tetany and spastic contractures of the arms were noticed in a 60-year-old man who had a radical neck dissection for invasive thyroid cancer

_____ 14. Pituitary tumor in a 30-year-old woman who ceased menstruating and began secreting milk

_____ 15. Weakness, dark pigmentation of skin, and hypotension in a man with tuberculosis. Corticosteroid levels in the blood were low, and corticotropin values were high.

_____ 16. Diabetes mellitus, porosity of bones, truncal obesity, and hypertension were diagnosed in a man with a radiologically enlarged sella turcica. Corticosteroid and corticotropin levels in the blood were high.

_____ 17. A 40-year-old woman complained of extensive sweating, tachycardia, and nervousness. She had bulging eyes and an enlarged thyroid. High blood levels of T_3 and T_4 were noted.

_____ 18. Myxedema and a hoarse voice

_____ 19. A 40-year-old woman complained of headaches, muscle weakness, menstrual irregularities, and visual disturbances. Prognathism, enlarged hands, and widened feet were present.

_____ 20. Bone deformities, calcification of soft tissues, and enlargement of all four parathyroids in a patient with chronic glomerulonephritis.

DIRECTIONS: Choose the one best answer.

_____ 21. Which is the most common pituitary tumor?
A. Corticotroph adenoma
B. Prolactinoma
C. Oncocytoma
D. Gonadotroph adenoma
E. Carcinoma

_____ 22. Most cases of thyroiditis are caused by
A. viruses.
B. bacteria.
C. parasites.
D. fungi.
E. autoimmune mechanisms.

_____ 23. Granulomatous inflammation of the thyroid and the presence of giant cells is typical of
A. Hashimoto thyroiditis.
B. Riedel thyroiditis.
C. lymphadenoid thyroiditis.
D. Graves disease.
E. subacute (DeQuervain) thyroiditis.

_____ 24. Thyroid cancer in a 30-year-old woman that metastasized to the regional lymph nodes most likely represents
A. papillary carcinoma.
B. follicular carcinoma.
C. oncocytic carcinoma.
D. medullary carcinoma.
E. undifferentiated carcinoma.

_____ 25. Which of the following histologic types of thyroid cancer has a tendency to be familial and occur as part of *MEN-2*?
A. Papillary
B. Follicular
C. Oncocytic
D. Medullary
E. Undifferentiated

_____ 26. Kidney stones are a complication of
A. hyperthyroidism.
B. hypothyroidism.
C. hyperparathyroidism.
D. hypoparathyroidism.
E. medullary carcinoma of the thyroid.

_____ 27. Tertiary hyperparathyroidism is a complication of
A. adrenal insufficiency.
B. renal insufficiency.
C. chronic malabsorption.
D. chronic diarrhea.
E. chronic liver disease.

_____ 28. Congenital deficiency of 21-hydroxylase ($P450_{c21}$) results in
A. Conn syndrome.
B. Cushing syndrome.
C. adrenogenital syndrome.
D. neonatal jaundice.
E. type I diabetes.

_____ 29. Hyperaldosteronism and increased blood renin are typical of
A. chronic adrenal failure.
B. chronic renal failure.
C. Conn syndrome.
D. Cushing syndrome.
E. adrenogenital syndrome.

_____ **30.** The most common cause of Cushing syndrome is
   A. exogenous corticosteroids.
   B. corticotropin-secreting pituitary adenoma.
   C. corticotropin-secreting lung cancer.
   D. adrenal cortical adenoma.
   E. adrenal cortical carcinoma.

A n s w e r s

1. **The answer is S.** The *syndrome of inappropriate ADH* secretion is characterized by massive retention of water. It is most often caused by secretion of ADH from small cell carcinoma of the lung.

2. **The answer is R.** *Sheehan syndrome* describes acute pituitary insufficiency, typically caused by infarction of the pituitary following delivery. The pituitary physiologically enlarges during pregnancy, and a sudden reduction in blood flow (e.g., due to massive postpartum bleeding) may cause ischemic necrosis.

3. **The answer is Q.** *Pheochromocytoma* is a tumor of the adrenal medulla that secretes epinephrine and norepinephrine. Release of these catecholamines occurs at irregular intervals, resulting in paroxysms of hypertension.

4. **The answer is G.** *Diabetes insipidus* is caused by head trauma that damages the posterior lobe of the pituitary (or the hypothalamus) and thus interrupts the secretion of the antidiuretic hormone (ADH). Lack of ADH results in excessive diuresis and polyuria.

5. **The answer is M.** *Cretinism* denotes mental insufficiency that is secondary to neonatal hypothyroidism. Compulsory iodination of salt has reduced the incidence of cretinism in the United States and other countries. The most common cause of neonatal hypothyroidism today is agenesis of the thyroid, which occurs at a rate of 1 in 4000 newborns.

6. **The answer is P.** *Neuroblastoma* is a malignant tumor of precursors of the adrenal medulla. These cells are derived from the neural crest and, like their more mature descendants in the adrenal medulla, may secrete catecholamines. These compounds are metabolized and excreted as vanillylmandelic acid in the urine.

7. **The answer is Q.** Although most *pheochromocytomas* originate from the adrenal medulla, some arise in sympathetic paraganglia. The neoplastic chromaffin cells exhibit granules that contain epinephrine and norepinephrine.

8. **The answer is B.** *Addison disease,* which presents with adrenal insufficiency, is most often caused by autoimmune adrenalitis.

9. **The answer is L.** *DiGeorge syndrome* is a developmental disorder of branchial clefts that is marked by agenesis of the parathyroids and thymus. It presents with signs of hypoparathyroidism (e.g., tetany) and defects in cell-mediated immunity.

10. **The answer is H.** *Multinodular goiter* is the most common cause of thyroid enlargement in middle-aged women. It is not usually associated

with functional disturbances and causes only cosmetic defects. In severe cases, it compresses the trachea, larynx, and other neck structures.

11. **The answer is F.** *Cushing syndrome* presents with an accumulation of subcutaneous fat on the posterior neck ("buffalo hump"), striae, and diabetes mellitus. In this case the disorder was caused by an adrenal tumor, which could have been either a cortical adenoma or carcinoma. These tumors secrete steroid hormones and are typically yellow on section.

12. **The answer is I.** *Primary hyperparathyroidism* presents as hypercalcemia and is most often caused by parathyroid adenoma.

13. **The answer is L.** *Hypoparathyroidism* results in tetany and spasms of skeletal muscles. In adults it is usually related to inadvertent removal of the parathyroids during thyroid surgery.

14. **The answer is D.** *Amenorrhea-galactorrhea* is a syndrome caused by pituitary tumors (prolactinomas), which impair menstruation and stimulate the secretion of milk.

15. **The answer is B.** *Addison disease*, or chronic adrenal insufficiency, was previously most often a complication of tuberculosis, which is still a common cause in underdeveloped countries. The disease presents with weakness, hypotension, anorexia and weight loss. Hyperpigmentation of the skin is caused by excess secretion of corticotropin by the pituitary.

16. **The answer is E.** *Cushing disease* is caused by pituitary tumors that secrete corticotropin. The disease presents with signs of adrenal hyperfunction. Dilatation enlargement of the sella turcica due to the pituitary adenoma is demonstrated radiologically. Both corticotropin and corticosteroid levels in the blood are elevated.

17. **The answer is K.** *Hyperthyroidism* presents with signs of hypermetabolism, such as sweating, tachycardia, and nervousness. In most instances it is caused by Graves disease, which is also characterized by exophthalmus. The thyroid is enlarged and warm. It secretes T_4 and T_3, the levels of which are elevated in the blood. Graves disease is an autimmune disease in which antibodies to TSH receptor act as agonists, thereby stimulating thyroid function.

18. **The answer is M.** *Myxedema* is a sign of hypothyroidism. Myxedematous patients have boggy facies, puffy eyelids, edema of extremities, and an enlarged tongue. The skin is pale, cold, and dry, owing to cutaneous vasoconstriction. The voice is hoarse because of laryngeal edema.

19. **The answer is A.** *Acromegaly* refers to enlargement of the terminal portions of the extremities and the jaw and is caused by growth hormone–secreting tumors of the pituitary. The pituitary tumor may lead to headaches and may compress the optic chiasm. These patients also have other hormonal problems, such as menstrual irregularities or diabetes mellitus.

20. **The answer is J.** *Secondary hyperparathyroidism* is a complication of chronic renal insufficiency. Excess parathyroid hormone causes renal osteodystrophy, or in severe cases, osteitis cystica fibrosa. The latter is characterized by severe bone deformities and the formation of "brown tumors of hyperparathyroidism."

21. **The answer is B.** *Prolactinomas* account for 25% of all pituitary tumors and thus represent the most common pituitary tumor.

22. The answer is E. Thyroiditis is in most instances an *autoimmune disease*.

23. The answer is E. *Subacute (DeQuervain) thyroiditis,* also known as *granulomatous thyroiditis,* is characterized by a granulomatous reaction and giant cells, which are a response to the rupture of thyroid follicles and leakage of colloid.

24. The answer is A. *Papillary carcinoma of the thyroid* is the most common thyroid tumor in younger women. It has a tendency to metastasize to regional lymph nodes, but distant metastases are rare. This tumor is usually cured by surgery.

25. The answer is D. *Medullary carcinoma of the thyroid* is often familial (*MEN-2A*) and occurs concomittantly with pheochromocytomas.

26. The answer is C. *Hyperparathyroidism* causes hypercalcemia, which may lead to the formation of renal stones.

27. The answer is B. *Tertiary hyperparathyroidism* is a complication of chronic renal failure. Enlarged parathyroid glands become independently hyperfunctional and must be removed surgically.

28. The answer is C. Congenital deficiency of 21-hydroxylase results in *adrenogenital syndrome,* which is associated with virilization of external genitalia in female infants (pseudohermaphroditism). Male infants show normal external genitalia. Hyponatremia, hyperkalemia, dehydration, and hypotension may develop, owing to inadequate synthesis of aldosterone.

29. The answer is B. Hyperreninemic hyperaldosteronism is usually caused by *renal disease,* which results in overstimulation of juxtaglomerular cells to secrete renin. Renin acts to stimulate aldosterone secretion by converting angiotensinogen to angiotensin. Primary aldosteronism (Conn syndrome) is associated with low or normal renin levels and is caused by tumors of zona glomerulosa of the adrenal cortex.

30. The answer is A. *Exogenous corticosteroids,* which are used to treat rheumatoid arthritis, nephrotic syndrome, asthma, and other diseases, are the most common cause of Cushing syndrome.

Diabetes

Questions

DIRECTIONS: Choose the one best answer.

_____ 1. Type I diabetes is characterized by all the following *except*
A. abrupt onset of polyuria and polydipsia.
B. low levels of insulin in the serum.
C. destruction of islets.
D. appearance of ketoacidosis in untreated patients.
E. high concordance in identical twins.

_____ 2. Type II diabetes is more common in
A. males than in females.
B. obese than in nonobese persons.
C. younger than in older persons.
D. taller than shorter persons.
E. blond than dark-haired persons.

_____ 3. Renal arteriolosclerosis of diabetes mellitus is caused by all the following *except*
A. polyuria.
B. arterial hypertension.
C. accumulation of basement membrane components.
D. glycosylation of cell wall components.
E. aggregation of platelets and decreased fibrinolysis.

_____ 4. Chronic ulcers on the feet of diabetic patients develop because of
A. abnormal glycosylation of hemoglobin.
B. inadequate leukocytic response to infection.
C. microvascular disease.
D. low concentrations of insulin in tissues.
E. increased incidence of varicose veins.

_____ 5. Renal complications of diabetes include all the following *except*
A. nodular glomerulosclerosis.
B. diffuse glomerular basement membrane thickening.
C. papillary necrosis.
D. fibrinoid necrosis of arcuate and interlobular arteries.
E. pyelonephritis.

_____ **6.** All the following are features of diabetic retinopathy *except*
  A. basement membrane thickening of capillaries.
  B. microaneurysms.
  C. retinal hemorrhages.
  D. proliferation of blood vessels and connective tissue.
  E. microabscesses.

DIRECTIONS: For each patient showing a complication of diabetes, select the most likely diagnosis.

Complications of Diabetes

  A. Atherosclerosis
  B. Cataract
  C. Glaucoma
  D. Hyaline arteriolosclerosis
  E. Nodular glomerulosclerosis
  F. Peripheral neuropathy
  G. Pyelonephritis, acute
  H. Pyelonephritis, chronic
  I. Renal papillary necrosis
  J. Retinopathy, nonproliferative
  K. Retinopathy, proliferative

_____ **7.** A 60-year-old man with a 10-year history of diabetes complained of deep burning pain and sensitivity to touch over his hands and fingers. Nerve conduction studies showed slow transmission of impulses.

_____ **8.** A 65-year-old man with a 20-year history of diabetes complained that he develops severe pain in his calves during walking.

_____ **9.** A 70-year-old diabetic complained of incontinence and inability to have an erection.

_____ **10.** A 30-year-old woman with a 10-year history of Type I diabetes noticed deteriorating eyesight. Funduscopic examination revealed numerous new blood vessels in the retina.

_____ **11.** A 50-year-old man known to have diabetes for 20 years developed generalized edema. He had 3$^+$ proteinuria and glucosuria. Serum albumin was 3 gm/dL, and serum cholesterol was 350 mg/dL. All other findings were within normal limits.

_____ **12.** A 60-year-old diabetic woman was hospitalized following an attack of renal colic. The ureter was found to be obstructed by a sloughed tip of a renal papilla.

_____ **13.** A 75-year-old woman with well-controlled diabetes complained of poor eyesight. A grayish white opacification of the lens was found on ophthalmoscopic examination.

_____ **14.** A 40-year-old woman who was 30 weeks pregnant with her fifth child developed diabetes and complained of flank pain radiating into the pelvis. She had fever (37.9°C) and the urinalysis revealed pyuria.

A n s w e r s

1. **The answer is E.** Type I diabetes is usually marked by the rapid onset of symptoms, such as polyuria and polydipsia. Ketoacidosis may develop early in untreated patients. The destruction of pancreatic islets is associated with *low blood insulin levels*, and replacement therapy with exogenous insulin is the only treatment presently available.

2. **The answer is B.** In contrast to type II diabetes, which shows a 90% concordance in identical twins, type I diabetes is discordant in 50%. Females are slightly more susceptible to type II diabetes than males. The disease is more common in *obese persons* than in those of normal weight. Type II diabetes is typically a disease of older people. Height or hair color is not linked to diabetes.

3. **The answer is A.** The pathogenesis of renal arteriolosclerosis in diabetes is not well understood. It seems to be a multifactorial disturbance, and all the factors listed except *polyuria* may play a role.

4. **The answer is C.** *Microvascular disease*, a characteristic of diabetes, causes ischemia and is in part responsible for the slow healing of wounds in the diabetic. The susceptibility of diabetics to infection is a complex problem, but it does not seem that the functions of polymorphonuclear leukocytes are directly affected. The tissue concentration of insulin does not influence the healing process. Diabetes does not predispose to varicose veins.

5. **The answer is D.** Glomerulosclerosis of diabetes occurs either in a nodular mesangial form (Kimmelstiel-Wilson disease) or as diffuse basement membrane thickening of the capillary loops. Papillary necrosis, an important complication of diabetes, is related to ischemia from microvascular disease and a susceptibility to pyelonephritis. Large blood vessels show atherosclerosis, but *fibrinoid necrosis* of muscular arteries, such as occurs in scleroderma and polyarteritis nodosa, is not seen in diabetes.

6. **The answer is E.** Diabetic retinopathy is associated with basement membrane changes, microaneurysms, retinal hemorrhages, and proliferation of retinal blood vessels. *Microabscesses* are not a feature of diabetic retinopathy.

7. **The answer is F.** *Peripheral sensory or sensory-motor neuropathy* is a common complication of diabetes. It is associated with demyelination—a loss of axons. It typically presents with a cramp or deep burning pain, cutaneous hyperesthesia, or insensitivity to changes of temperature. Touch and vibratory sense may be reduced. Changes in nerve conduction are usually a sign of advanced irreversible changes.

8. **The answer is A.** Leg pain during walking or exercise, which forces the patient to stop or limp (claudication), is typically a complication of *atherosclerosis* involving the major arteries of the lower extremities.

9. **The answer is F.** Incontinence and erectile dysfunction of diabetics are related to *peripheral neuropathy* involving the autonomic nerves.

10. **The answer is K.** *New blood vessel formation in the retina* typically affects persons suffering from type I diabetes.

11. **The answer is E.** Edema, proteinuria, hypoalbuminemia, and hyperlipidemia are features of nephrotic syndrome, secondary to the glomerular changes in patients with longstanding diabetes. Glomerular changes occur in two forms, namely, diffuse or *nodular glomerulosclerosis* (Kimmelstiel-Wilson disease).

12. **The answer is I.** Renal *papillary necrosis* is caused by severe ischemia of the renal medulla, which may occur in patients with severe diabetic microangiopathy. The necrotic papillae may slough off into the ureters, causing obstruction and renal colic.

13. **The answer is B.** *Cataract* (i.e., opacification of the lens) is a common disease of old age that occurs with increased frequency in patients with diabetes. These cataracts may be related to the metabolic changes typically found in diabetes, although their exact pathogenesis is not understood.

14. **The answer is G.** Flank pain, fever, and pyuria are indicative of *acute pyelonephritis*, a common complication of diabetes. The symptoms of chronic pyelonephritis are usually less obvious, and urinalysis does not always provide proof of infection.

Chapter 23

Amyloidosis

Questions

DIRECTIONS: Match each numbered statement with the most appropriate lettered item. Each lettered item can be used once, more than once, or not at all.

Forms of Amyloid

    A. AA Amyloid
    B. AE Amyloid
    C. AL Amyloid
    D. β-amyloid
    E. β_2-microglobulin
    F. Isolated atrial amyloid
    G. Prion amyloid
    H. Transthyretin-derived amyloid

_____ 1. Familial Mediterranean fever

_____ 2. Intraneural deposits of amyloid in familial amyloidotic polyneuropathy

_____ 3. Deposits of amyloid in the brain in Alzheimer disease

_____ 4. Cerebral deposits of amyloid in Down syndrome

_____ 5. Pancreatic islets in diabetes mellitus

_____ 6. Senile cardiac amyloidosis

_____ 7. Nephrotic syndrome in multiple myeloma

_____ 8. Bronchiectasis with chronic suppuration

_____ 9. Chronic suppurative osteomyelitis

_____ 10. Medullary carcinoma of the thyroid

_____ 11. Amyloidosis in patients undergoing hemodialysis

_____ 12. Amyloidosis as a paraneoplastic complication of renal cell carcinoma

_____ 13. Amyloidosis in Hodgkin's disease

_____ 14. Amyloidosis in B-cell lymphoma

_____ **15.** Interleukin-1 stimulates the liver to synthesize the precursor of this amyloid.

_____ **16.** Cardiac amyloid derived from atrial natriuretic polypeptide

A n s w e r s

1. **The answer is A.** Familial Mediterranean fever is an autosomal recessive disease that predominantly affects Sephardic Jews, Arabs, Turks, and Armenians. It is characterized by chronic and recurrent infections, owing to the dysfunction of leukocytes. Similar to any other suppurative inflammation, this disease promotes the synthesis of serum *amyloid A* (SAA) protein. SAA released from the liver into the blood is converted into AA amyloid, which is then deposited in many organs, as in secondary amyloidosis caused by other nonfamilial forms of chronic suppurative inflammation.

2. **The answer is H.** Familial amyloidotic polyneuropathy is an autosomal dominant disorder that affects families in Sweden, Portugal, and Japan and is related to a mutation in the *transthyretin* gene. Amyloid in the peripheral and autonomic nerves is derived from the abnormal transthyretin.

3. **The answer is D.** Amyloid deposits in the brain and cerebral vessels of patients suffering from Alzheimer disease contain fibrils of *β-amyloid*. This 4-kD protein is encoded by a gene on chromosome 21.

4. **The answer is D.** Brains of middle-aged patients with Down syndrome show changes similar to those of Alzheimer disease. As in Alzheimer disease, the deposits of cerebral amyloid are derived from *β-amyloid*.

5. **The answer is B.** In diabetes mellitus type II, the islets of Langerhans often contain *amyloid AE*. This amyloid is derived from amylin, also known as islet amyloid polypeptide, a hormone closely related to calcitonin.

6. **The answer is H.** Senile cardiac amyloid is derived from *transthyretin*. Cardiac deposits of amyloid occur most often in men over 70 years of age, who are usually asymptomatic. Massive deposits, especially in younger men, may cause heart failure.

7. **The answer is C.** Multiple myeloma is accompanied by amyloidosis in 10% to 15% of cases. The amyloid fibrils consist of *AL amyloid*, which is derived from the variable region of the kappa or lambda light chains of immunoglobulin. Accordingly, the composition of AL amyloid varies from one patient to another.

8. **The answer is A.** Chronic bronchiectasis may be accompanied by deposits of *AA amyloid*. This secondary amyloidosis most often affects the kidneys, liver, adrenals, and spleen.

9. **The answer is A.** Chronic suppurative osteomyelitis is accompanied by secondary amyloidosis, characterized by deposits of *AA amyloid*.

10. **The answer is B.** The stroma of medullary carcinoma of the thyroid contains deposits of *AE amyloid* derived from precalcitonin.

11. **The answer is E.** Deposits of amyloid in patients on chronic hemodialysis consist of β_2-*microglobulin*. Amyloid is typically found in the joints and gastrointestinal tract.

12. **The answer is A.** Renal cell carcinoma is occasionally accompanied by secondary amyloidosis. These deposits consist of *AA amyloid*.

13. **The answer is A.** Hodgkin's disease may be complicated by amyloidosis. Deposits consist of *AA amyloid*.

14. **The answer is C.** Amyloid found in patients suffering from B-cell lymphoma is of *AL type*. Similar to amyloid of multiple myeloma these fibrils are derived from the variable portion of the immunoglobulin light chain.

15. **The answer is A.** Serum amyloid A (SAA), the precursor of *AA amyloid*, is secreted by the liver as an acute-phase reactant, typically in response to acute inflammation. Interleukin 1 is a potent stimulator of SAA synthesis.

16. **The answer is F.** *Isolated atrial amyloid* is derived from atrial natriuretic polypeptide.

Chapter 24

The Skin

Questions

DIRECTIONS: Match each numbered statement with the most appropriate lettered item. Each lettered item can be used once, more than once, or not at all.

Skin Lesions

    A. Alopecia
    B. Blister
    C. Comedo
    D. Macule
    E. Nodule
    F. Papule
    G. Plaque
    H. Pustule
    I. Ulcer
    J. Wheal

_____ 1. Typical early lesion of herpes simplex virus infection
_____ 2. Freckle (ephelis)
_____ 3. Psoriasis
_____ 4. Vertical growth phase melanoma
_____ 5. Syphilitic chancre
_____ 6. Impetigo
_____ 7. Verruca vulgaris
_____ 8. Hair loss caused by chemotherapy
_____ 9. "Blackheads" of acne vulgaris
_____ 10. Urticaria

Skin Diseases

    A. Acne vulgaris
    B. Acute eczematous dermatitis

C. Allergic contact dermatitis
D. Bullous pemphigoid
E. Dermatitis herpetiformis
F. Epidermolysis bullosa
G. Erythema multiforme
H. Erythema nodosum
I. Ichthyosis vulgaris
J. Hypersensitivity angiitis
K. Lichen planus
L. Lupus erythematosus
M. Pemphigus vulgaris
N. Psoriasis
O. Scleroderma
P. Tinea corporis
Q. Urticaria pigmentosa

_____ 11. A 3-year-old child had numerous small, white scales covering the extensor surfaces of the extremities, trunk, and face. The skin biopsy showed hyperkeratosis, which was disproportionate to the thin stratum spongiosum.

_____ 12. A 20-year-old man had numerous plaques covered with pearly scales over the elbows, face, and scalp. A skin biopsy showed clublike elongation of epidermal rete pegs and reciprocal upward extension of dermal papillae. The latter contained dilated vessels and inflammatory cells that extended into the thin overlying epidermis. The epidermis was covered with thick layers of keratin, with focal parakeratosis.

_____ 13. A 25-year-old man suffered periodic eruptions of blisters on the scalp and inner surface of the groin, and in the mouth. Histologically, the lesions showed separation of the stratum spinosum from the basal layer. Linear deposits of antibodies were demonstrated by indirect immunofluorescence microscopy on the surface of the epidermal cell.

_____ 14. Numerous blisters were found on the trunk and extremities of a 2-day-old neonate. Skin biopsy disclosed separation of the basal layer of the epidermis from its basement membrane. No inflammatory cells or antibody deposits were seen.

_____ 15. Large blisters appeared on the flexor surfaces of the forearms of a 60-year-old woman. Skin biopsy showed separation of the basal layer of the epidermis from the basement membrane. Linear deposits of IgG and C3 complement were detected in the basement membrane.

_____ 16. A 15-year-old woman with gluten sensitivity developed itchy, wheal-like lesions, with small vesicles over the elbows and knees. A skin biopsy revealed inflammation in the tips of the dermal papillae and subepidermal vesicles. Deposits of IgA were seen in the dermal papillae by immunofluorescence microscopy.

_____ 17. A 20-year-old woman complained of joint pain and skin rash on sun-exposed areas of the face, neck, and chest. A skin biopsy revealed vacuolar change in the basal layer of epidermis, thickening of the basement membrane, hyperkeratotic plugging of the follicles, and a lymphocytic inflammatory infiltrate in the dermis. Granular deposits of IgG and C3 complement were present along the epidermal basement membrane by immunofluorescence microscopy.

_____ 18. Violaceous, flat-topped papules appeared gradually on the flexor surfaces of the wrists of a 30-year-old man. White streaks and patches were also found on the buccal mucosa of the mouth. Histologically, the lesions showed hyperkeratosis, thickening of the stratum granulosum, and a bandlike infiltrate of lymphocytes and macrophages in the upper dermis, disrupting the basal layer of the epidermis. Lymphocytes were mostly of the CD4 type.

_____ 19. Purpuric, 2- to 4-mm papules appeared on the skin of a 28-year-old woman. The papules did not blanch under pressure. Histologically, the dermis showed necrotizing leukocytoclastic venulitis.

_____ 20. Dome-shaped erythematous nodules suddenly appeared on the skin of a 28-year-old woman. A skin biopsy disclosed focal hemorrhage, neutrophilic infiltrates in the subcutaneous fibrous tissue septa, and giant cells at the interface between the septa and the adipose fat tissue. No infectious agents were identified.

_____ 21. A 20-year-old man presented to his family physician for treatment of what he said was "a severe attack of poison ivy." The patient's hands and arms appeared red and were covered with oozing blisters and crusts.

_____ 22. A 40-year-old woman noticed stiffness of skin over the fingers and nonpitting edema. The skin of the face had also become tense, and around the mouth it showed radial furrows. A skin biopsy showed collagen bundles parallel to an atrophic epidermis, together with a loss of dermal appendages.

DIRECTIONS: Match the following numbered words or sentences with the most appropriate dermatopathologic diagnosis.

Tumors and Tumorlike Lesions of the Skin

A. Acanthosis nigricans
B. Actinic keratosis
C. Basal cell carcinoma
D. Benign fibrous histiocytoma
E. Epithelial inclusion cyst
F. Fibroepithelial polyp
G. Freckle (ephelis)
H. Hemangioma
I. Histiocytosis X
J. Kaposi sarcoma
K. Keratoacanthoma
L. Lentigo
M. Malignant melanoma
N. Mastocytosis

O. Melanoma
P. Mycosis fungoides
Q. Nevus
R. Seborrheic keratosis
S. Skin appendix tumors
T. Squamous cell carcinoma
U. Xanthoma

_____ **23.** A rodent ulcer on the lateral side of the nose. Histologically, it was composed of basaloid cells forming solid nests with peripheral palisading.

_____ **24.** A 3-cm indurated and ulcerated nodule on the back of the forearm. Histologically, it was composed of infiltrating nests of atypical keratinizing epithelium. The tumor cells formed intercellular bridges and keratin "pearls."

_____ **25.** A dark red nodule on the chest of a 30-year-old homosexual, HIV-positive man. Histologically, the lesion was composed of indistinct vascular spaces filled with red blood cells.

_____ **26.** Skin nodules composed of neoplastic T cells were found in a 60-year-old man.

_____ **27.** An 80-year-old farmer developed 1-cm, red, slightly raised plaque on the face. Histologically, it showed cytologic atypia and dyskeratosis, limited to the basal layers of the stratum spongiosum, hyperkeratosis, and parakeratosis.

_____ **28.** A 28-year-old woman noticed a 2-mm dark dot on her chest, which slowly became darker and enlarged over a period of 2 years to a size of 4 mm.

DIRECTIONS: Match the following suggested diagnoses with the most appropriate lettered part of Figure 24-1. Each lettered part can be used once, more than once, or not at all.

_____ **29.** Basal cell carcinoma
_____ **30.** Squamous cell carcinoma
_____ **31.** Melanoma
_____ **32.** Kaposi sarcoma

A n s w e r s

1. **The answer is B.** Herpes simplex virus (HSV) causes small grouped *blisters* on the skin or the mucosa. Small blisters measuring less than 5 mm in diameter are called *vesicles*; larger ones are termed *bullae*. Secondary bacterial infection may transform herpetic vesicles into pustules.

2. **The answer is D.** Freckles are small, pigmented *macules* (i.e., flat areas of altered pigmentation in light-skinned persons). Freckles typically appear in children after exposure to the sun and fade in winter. Histologically, such lesions consist of keratinocytes laden with melanin.

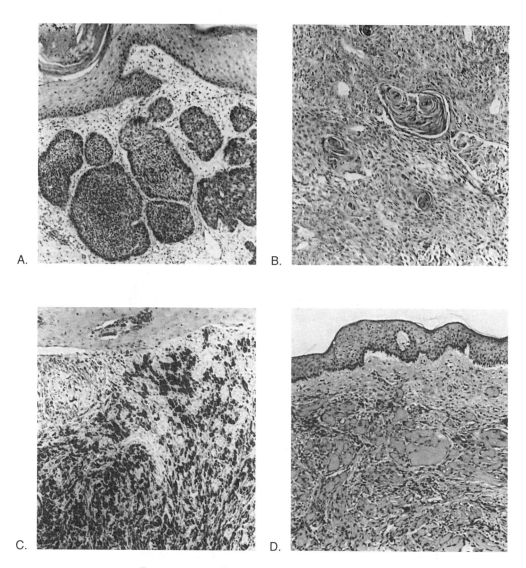

FIGURE 24-1. HISTOLOGY OF SKIN NEOPLASMS.

3. **The answer is G.** Psoriasis is a chronic disease that presents with numerous erythematous, scaly *plaques*. These plaques consist of a thickened epidermis showing keratosis and parakeratosis, and marked elongation of rete ridges.

4. **The answer is E.** Malignant melanoma in the vertical growth phase invades the dermis and forms a *nodule* (i.e., discrete solid mass extending below the epidermis and protruding above it).

5. **The answer is I.** A syphilitic chancre is an *ulcer* (i.e., a defect of the epidermis). It occurs typically on the mucosa or skin of the male and female external genitalia.

6. **The answer is H.** Impetigo contagiosa, a skin infection typically caused by *Staphylococcus aureus* presents with *pustules* (i.e., pus-containing vesicles or papules).

7. **The answer is F.** Verruca vulgaris (common wart) presents as a *papule* or a slightly raised skin lesion less than 5 mm in diameter. Histologically, a wart consists of a thickened epidermis (acanthosis) showing hyperkeratosis and thickening of the granular layer. Human papilloma virus (HPV) is present in the keratinocytes.

8. **The answer is A.** Alopecia, or hair loss, due to chemotherapy is diffuse but temporary.

9. **The answer is C.** *Comedos,* or "blackheads," are typical lesions of acne vulgaris. They represent distended follicles filled with oxidized sebum and keratin that are prone to infection with the anaerobic diphtheroid *Propionobacterium acnes.*

10. **The answer is J.** *Wheals* are evanescent, edematous papules or plaques that are typical lesions of urticaria. Urticaria are characterized by localized edema of skin and are often a sign of type I hypersensitivity reaction, in which case they are caused by IgE-related degranulation of dermal mast cells. However, wheals may result from IgE-independent degranulation of mast cells, caused by physical factors (as in dermatographism), chemicals, and drugs, or by complement activation (hereditary angioneurotic edema).

11. **The answer is I.** *Ichthyosis vulgaris* is the most common of the ichthyoses, a group of diseases characterized by excessive keratinization. It begins in childhood and is often hereditary. The disease is not curable but the skin can be maintained free of scales with topical treatment.

12. **The answer is N.** *Psoriasis* is a disease of unknown etiology characterized by the periodic appearance of plaques covered with silvery scales on the skin overlying the elbows, knees, intertriginous areas, and the scalp. Hair loss, involvement of the nails, and arthritis are found in some patients. It is thought that abnormal proliferation and maturation of epidermal cells and an abnormal vascular response in the papillary dermis are related to the pathogenesis of psoriasis.

13. **The answer is M.** *Pemphigus vulgaris* is an autoimmune disease characterized by the binding of antibodies to an epidermal cell surface antigen, which causes their dissociation from the basal layer and leads to the formation of suprabasal bullae. Bullae occur most often on mucosal surfaces, the scalp, and periumbilical and intertriginous skin.

14. **The answer is F.** *Epidermolysis bullosa* is a group of diseases, all of which are characterized by an appearance of blisters at birth or shortly thereafter. These conditions are caused by mutations in genes encoding the adhesion and cytoskeletal proteins that join the epidermal cells. Minor mechanical trauma, such as rubbing, may blister the epidermis, which, however, heals without scarring.

15. **The answer is D.** *Bullous pemphigoid* is an autoimmune disease of older persons characterized by the deposition of autoantibodies in the basement membrane of the epidermis. These antibodies cause dermal/epidermal separation, with the formation of subepidermal vesicles and bullae. The blisters appear on the medial aspects of the thighs and the flexor aspects of forearms but may also occur in other sites.

16. **The answer is E.** *Dermatitis herpetiformis* is an autoimmune disease characterized by hypersensitivity to gluten and deposition of IgA in dermal papillae. The autoantibodies cause dermal inflammation and the formation of small vesicles resembling those seen in herpesvirus infection (herpetiform).

17. **The answer is L.** *Lupus erythematosus* is an autoimmune disease typically presenting with dermatitis on sun-exposed areas, arthritis, and nephritis. The malady features the deposition of immune complexes along the epidermal/dermal junction and is accompanied by inflammation of the dermis, particularly prominent around hair follicles and blood vessels.

18. **The answer is K.** *Lichen planus* is a disease of unknown etiology, often associated with other diseases such as ulcerative colitis or exposure to drugs and chemicals. Scaly papules (lichenoid eruption) of the skin and mucosal surfaces are composed of T-helper lymphocytes invading the epidermis.

19. **The answer is J.** *Palpable purpura* that does not fade upon compression is typical of *hypersensitivity angiitis*. This reaction reflects the deposition of antigen/autoantibody complexes in the walls of small blood vessels, with subsequent necrotizing inflammation. Antibodies may form in response to viral infections (e.g., hepatitis B virus) or drugs, but the antigen usually remains unknown.

20. **The answer is H.** *Erythema nodosum* is a self-limited disease that presents with subcutaneous nodules on the extensor surfaces of the lower extremities. It is related to infections or exposure to drugs, but its precise pathogenesis remains unknown. It is thought that neutrophils appear in the connective-tissue septa of the dermis in response to deposits of activated complement proteins. Macrophages and giant cells probably represent a reaction to fat necrosis caused by acute inflammation.

21. **The answer is C.** "Poison ivy" is a type IV hypersensitivity reaction to plants of the *Rhus* genus. This T-cell-mediated *allergic contact dermatitis* presents as urticaria and bullous eruption. Blisters rupture and heal with crusts, usually without scarring.

22. **The answer is O.** *Scleroderma* is an autoimmune disorder of unknown etiology characterized by progressive thickening of the dermis. It is four times more common in women than in men, and its peak incidence is in the 30- to 50-year age group. Collagen of the dermis becomes abnormally sclerotic, causing atrophy of the epidermis and loss of skin appendages. Internal organs (e.g., esophagus, intestines, and lungs) may also be affected.

23. **The answer is C.** *Basal cell carcinoma* often presents as a pearly papule that tends to ulcerate with time and produce a "rodent ulcer." The tumor is composed of nests of deeply basophilic small cells, resembling those in the basal layer of the normal epidermis.

24. **The answer is T.** *Squamous cell carcinoma* is an invasive malignant tumor that occurs on sun-exposed areas of the skin. It appears as a nodule, which usually ulcerates. The tumor cells form strands extending into the dermis and subcutis. The tumor cells tend to retain features of squamous cells and undergo keratinization, forming so-called keratin pearls.

25. **The answer is J.** *Kaposi sarcoma* presents with hemorrhagic nodules that vary in size and color and may be red, brown, or bluish-black. These tumors are composed of blood-filled spaces lined by endothelial cells.

26. **The answer is P.** *Mycosis fungoides* is a neoplastic cutaneous disorder in which malignant T-lymphocytes infiltrate the skin, forming patches and nodules.

27. **The answer is B.** *Actinic keratosis* is a preinvasive carcinoma of the epidermis in which the atypical neoplastic cells are confined to the epidermis and do not invade through the basement membrane into the dermis. These lesions are typically found on sun-exposed skin.

28. **The answer is Q.** *Nevus*, or mole, is a skin hamartoma composed of pigmented nevus cells. Acquired nevi appear during early adulthood and usually involute spontaneously, supporting the dictum that most of us are born without nevi and die without them. Transformation of nevi into malignant melanoma occasionally occurs. In this circumstance the pigmented lesion usually enlarges, becomes irregularly shaped, and shows variation in pigmentation from one area to another.

29. **The answer is A.** *Basal cell carcinoma* is composed of small, uniform cells, forming nests that show palisading at their periphery.

30. **The answer is B.** *Squamous cell carcinoma* features sheets of epidermoid cells, which show central keratinization in the form of concentric whorls (keratin pearls).

31. **The answer is C.** *Melanoma* cells contain pigment (melanin) that may be shed from tumor cells and taken up by macrophages in the surrounding tissue.

32. **The answer is D.** *Kaposi sarcoma* is composed of blood-filled spaces lined by neoplastic endothelial cells.

The Head and Neck

Questions

DIRECTIONS: Match each numbered statement with the most appropriate lettered item. Each lettered item can be used once, more than once, or not at all.

Oral Lesions

A. Acute necrotizing ulcerative gingivitis (Vincent angina)
B. Aphthous stomatitis
C. Apical granuloma
D. Dental caries
E. Hairy leukoplakia
F. Herpes labialis
G. Ludwig angina
H. Periodontitis
I. Pulpitis
J. Pyogenic granuloma
K. Thrush
L. Xerostomia

_____ **1.** A 6-year-old boy had "flu" for a week. As soon as the fever subsided he developed small vesicles on the upper lip. The fluid of the vesicles contained multinucleated cells with ground-glass-like nuclear inclusions.

_____ **2.** A 60-year-old man with a 15-year history of diabetes was hospitalized because of end-stage kidney disease. His tongue, inner side of the lips, and buccal mucosa were covered with white, slightly elevated, soft patches, which could be easily scraped away. Microscopically, this material contained pseudohyphae and yeasts.

_____ **3.** A 40-year-old woman was hospitalized because of a massive neck infection that developed over a period of 3 days following extraction of an impacted wisdom tooth. She had a high fever and her lower jaw and entire neck were swollen, red, and painful. Throat culture revealed a mixed bacterial flora, containing both aerobic and anaerobic microorganisms.

_____ **4.** A 40-year-old woman with bilateral retromandibular neck masses complained of dryness of her mouth and eyes. On biopsy the neck masses were found to be enlarged salivary glands that were infiltrated with polyclonal lymphocytes, forming focal germinal centers. Benign lymphoepithelial lesions were also present.

_____ **5.** A 3-year-old girl was enrolled in a day care center but had to be withdrawn because she developed extensive, painful, superficial ulcers of the mouth. The ulcerations healed spontaneously over a period of 5 days.

_____ **6.** A soft red mass measuring 1 cm in diameter was surgically removed from the buccal gingiva of a 6-year-old boy. The lesion had a smooth external surface and was histologically composed of vascular spaces lined by angioblasts and surrounded by loose connective stroma infiltrated with neutrophils, lymphocytes, and plasma cells.

_____ **7.** A 60-year-old chronic alcoholic man was referred to the dentist for the treatment of punched-out gingival ulcers. The gingiva was focally covered with grayish-white layers of friable material that could be scraped away, leaving behind a red, bleeding surface.

_____ **8.** A 38-year-old man known to have AIDS complained of mouth soreness. Oral examination revealed confluent white patches on the mucosa. Microscopically the lesions were composed of layers of keratotic squamous cells and some koilocytic cells. No fungi could be identified.

_____ **9.** A 30-year-old man was told by his dentist that his left upper wisdom tooth showed some decay. Even though the decay was still reparable, he recommended that the tooth be extracted.

_____ **10.** A 24-year-old man woke up early because of excruciating pain in his lower jaw. His dentist told him that the inside of one of his teeth contained pus but fortunately did not extend into the jawbone.

_____ **11.** A 50-year-old man was told that he needed extensive treatment of his gum disease. He had "large pockets around his teeth" and his gums were inflamed.

_____ **12.** A 30-year-old man sought emergency treatment for throbbing pain in his upper jaw. X-rays showed a tooth infection that had spread into the jaw and locally destroyed the bone. The pathologist reported that material from the jaw consisted of acutely and chronically inflamed granulation tissue, with some fragments of normal squamous epithelium.

DIRECTIONS: Match each numbered statement with the most appropriate lettered diagnosis. Each lettered item can be used once, more than once, or not at all.

Diseases of the Nose, Nasopharynx, Larynx, Paranasal Sinuses, and Middle Ear

A. Acute rhinitis
B. Acute serous otitis media
C. Acute suppurative otitis media
D. Acute tonsillitis
E. Adenoids
F. Chronic serous otitis media
G. Chronic sinusitis
H. Chronic suppurative otitis media
I. Papilloma
J. Peritonsillar abscess ("quinsy")
K. Wegener granulomatosis

_____ **13.** "Runny nose" caused by viruses

_____ **14.** The most common cause of nonneoplastic polyps

_____ **15.** Nasal necrotizing granulomatous lesion commonly associated with pulmonary and renal lesions

_____ **16.** Wartlike lesion in the larynx caused by human papilloma virus

_____ **17.** A typical feature of "strep throat" but may also be caused by viruses

_____ **18.** Chronic inflammatory hyperplasia of lymphoid tissue in the posterior pharynx

_____ **19.** Bacterial infection that may have life-threatening consequences if unrecognized

_____ **20.** May be caused by deep-sea diving

_____ **21.** In adults it may be the initial sign of nasopharyngeal carcinoma

_____ **22.** Perforation of the eardrum caused by recent *Streptococcus pneumoniae* infection

_____ **23.** Cholesteatoma is a complication of this disease

Tumors of the Oral Cavity and Salivary Glands, Nose, and Nasopharynx

A. Adenoid cystic carcinoma
B. Adenolymphoma (Warthin tumor)
C. Ameloblastoma
D. Angiofibroma
E. Burkitt lymphoma
F. Mucoepidermoid carcinoma
G. Nasopharyngeal carcinoma
H. Papilloma
I. Peripheral giant cell granuloma

J. Pleomorphic adenoma
K. Squamous cell carcinoma

_____ **24.** Tumor arising from developmental rests of the enamel organ in the mandible

_____ **25.** Nonencapsulated mesenchymal tumor of the nasopharynx in a young man that responds well to radiation therapy

_____ **26.** A malignant tumor that is more common in China than in the United States

_____ **27.** A malignant tumor composed of keratin-positive cells embedded in lymphoid tissue

_____ **28.** An oral lesion that is also known as "epulis" or "osteoclastoma"

_____ **29.** A tumor that may present as oral leukoplakia

_____ **30.** The most common malignant tumor of the oral cavity, which is often multifocal

_____ **31.** A jaw tumor that occurs in an epidemic form in sub-Saharan Africa

_____ **32.** The most common salivary gland tumor, most often found in the parotid

Answers

1. **The answer is F.** Confluent vesicles that appear on the lips after or during an infection are typical of herpesvirus infection. *Herpes labialis* is caused by HSV type I. The virus can be identified in the nuclei of infected squamous cells in the vesicle fluid. By light microscopy the infected cells are multinucleated and have a ground-glass appearance.

2. **The answer is K.** White plaques in the mouth of chronically ill, immunosuppressed, or debilitated persons represent *thrush*. The lesions are caused by *Candida albicans*, a fungus that can be readily identified microscopically in the scraped material from the lesions.

3. **The answer is G.** Massive infection of the neck ("phlegmon") occurs in some patients following oral surgery and is called *Ludwig angina*. This infection is caused by a variety of bacterial pathogens, and the bacteriologic studies usually reveal a mixed bacterial flora. Immunosuppressed or debilitated patients are more prone to develop this potentially lethal form of infection, but it may also affect those who do not have any obvious risk factors. The infection may dissect through the anatomic planes of the neck between the muscles and neck organs and extend into the mediastinum.

4. **The answer is L.** Dryness of the mouth (xerostomia) and of the eye (xerophthalmia) are features of Sjögren syndrome. This autoimmune disease causes sialadenitis and dacryocystitis, destroying the secretory parts of salivary and lacrimal glands. Histologically, these glands are infiltrated with lymphocytes. The lymphocytic infiltrate may contain remaining ducts, which are known as *lymphoepithelial lesions*.

5. **The answer is B.** Superficial oral ulcers of sudden onset are features of *aphthous stomatitis*. These lesions, also known as aphthae or canker sores, heal spontaneously. The cause of aphthous stomatitis is unknown.

6. **The answer is J.** Small red nodules on the gingiva of children usually represent *pyogenic granulomas*. These lesions are highly vascular, and some pathologists consider them to be inflamed hemangiomas. Others believe them to represent hyperplastic granulation tissue and classify them as inflammatory rather than as neoplastic.

7. **The answer is A.** Punched-out ulcerations of interdental papillae and more extensive ulcerations covered with pseudomembranes are typical of *acute necrotizing ulcerative gingivitis* (Vincent angina). This lesion is caused by symbiotic action of a fusiform bacillus and a spirochete (*Borrelia vincentii*). Because these bacteria are normally found in the mouth, some predisposing factor must play a role in the pathogenesis of the lesions.

8. **The answer is E.** Some patients with AIDS develop *hairy leukoplakia*, a lesion that presents in the form of florid, whitish-gray plaques on the oral mucosa. The plaques contain squamous cells with signs of human papillomavirus infection.

9. **The answer is D.** Tooth decay is technically called *dental caries*.

10. **The answer is I.** Purulent infection of the inside of a tooth is called *pulpitis*. Bacteria enter the pulp cavity through defects of dentin that has been eroded by caries.

11. **The answer is H.** *Periodontitis* is caused by the accumulation of bacteria under the gingiva in periodontal pockets and is the main form of gum disease in adults. If not treated, this infection (caused by *Bacteroides gingivalis* and some other pathogens) results in the loss of teeth.

12. **The answer is C.** Tooth-related cavities of the jawbone may represent cysts, apical granulomas, or abscesses. Cysts are typically lined by squamous or dentigerous epithelium and may or may not be infected. So-called *apical granulomas* are actually composed of granulation tissue and are not true granulomas. They may contain foci of invaginated squamous epithelium. An abscess can form on its own or inside an apical granuloma or cyst. In this case an abscess formed in a preexisting apical granuloma.

13. **The answer is A.** *Acute rhinitis* is usually caused by viruses but may also be due to allergy. By contrast, chronic rhinitis is generally allergic.

14. **The answer is G.** Polyps are most often a consequence of *chronic sinusitis*. Allergy may cause sinusitis, but bacterial infection is often superimposed.

15. **The answer is K.** *Wegener granulomatosis* is a disease of unknown origin that shares some features with lethal midline granuloma. Both diseases are characterized by necrotizing, ulcerated, mucosal lesions. Lethal midline granuloma is a sign of an underlying lymphoid malignancy, whereas Wegener granulomatosis is an inflammatory disease. Evidence points to an autoimmune etiology for Wegener granulomatosis. In most instances the lesions are not limited to the upper respiratory tract; they also involve the lungs and the kidneys.

16. **The answer is I.** *Papillomas* may be histologically diagnosed as either squamous or inverted and are the most common tumors of the nasal cavity. Histologically, they are similar to warts.

17. **The answer is D.** *Acute tonsillitis* is usually caused by bacterial or viral infections. Among the bacterial ones, *Streptococcus pyogenes* is the most common etiologic agent.

18. **The answer is E.** *Adenoids* are "glandlike" enlargements of chronically inflamed lymphoid tissue in the posterior pharynx. Enlarged lymphoid tissue may obstruct the eustachian tube and cause otitis media or may interfere with breathing.

19. **The answer is J.** Quinsy, or *peritonsillar abscess,* results from inadequately treated bacterial tonsillitis. The pus from the abscess may extend into the upper or lower neck, or mediastinum, or even into the cranial cavity, with life-threatening consequences.

20. **The answer is B.** *Acute serous otitis media,* characterized by the accumulation of serous fluid in the middle ear, is caused by low external pressure. This is most often due to a sudden change in atmospheric pressure, as encountered in deep-sea diving or unpressurized airplane flights at high altitude.

21. **The answer is F.** *Chronic* or recurrent *serous otitis media* suggests a local cause, such as occlusion of the eustachian tube. In children, a common cause is adenoids, but in adults, one should consider the possibility of nasopharyngeal carcinoma.

22. **The answer is C.** *Streptococcus pneumoniae* is the most common infectious cause of *acute suppurative otitis,* a condition often complicated by perforation of the eardrum.

23. **The answer is H.** Cholesteatoma is a complication of *chronic suppurative otitis* and a rupture of the eardrum. It is an epidermal inclusion cyst formed by the epithelium that has grown into the middle ear through the perforation. Cholesteatomas tend to enlarge, either because the lining cells continue to grow or because the cysts become infected. Enlargement and secondary changes in the cholesteatoma cause erosion of the mastoid bone, auditory ossicles, and nerves, thereby aggravating the hearing loss and causing chronic pain. Cholesteatomas may be confused with neoplasms.

24. **The answer is C.** *Ameloblastomas* are tumors derived from odontogenic epithelium; they usually occur in the ramus or the molar area of the mandible. Histologically, as the name implies, the tumor is composed of ameloblasts that form islands resembling the enamel organ. It is therefore assumed that the tumor originates from a developmental rest of the enamel organ that has been retained in the jaw.

25. **The answer is D.** *Angiofibromas* are nonencapsulated tumors typically located in the nasopharynx of adolescent males. Radiation therapy gives excellent results and is preferred to surgery in the treatment of these vascular lesions.

26. **The answer is G.** *Nasopharyngeal carcinomas* are more common in Chinese than in other ethnic groups, suggesting a racially determined genetic susceptibility. Both the tumor cells and infiltrating lymphoid

cells frequently contain the Epstein-Barr virus. The role of the virus and its pathogenetic relationship to the tumor has not been elucidated.

27. **The answer is G.** *Nasopharyngeal carcinomas* are composed of large, atypical tumor cells intermixed with lymphoid cells. Their epithelial origin has been established by the immunohistochemical demonstration of keratin, desmosomes, and epithelial membrane antigen.

28. **The answer is I.** *Peripheral giant cell granuloma* is known by several names, such as epulis (Greek, "gumboil"), osteoclastoma, or giant cell tumor of the gum. These lesions are more likely reactive than neoplastic. Histologically, the lesion consists of numerous blood vessels, fibroblasts, and giant cells. Although giant cells resemble osteoclasts, their derivation has not been elucidated. Peripheral, giant cell, reparative granulomas are indistinguishable from giant cell lesions of bone (called "central") or from the "brown tumors" of hyperparathyroidism. The latter are also hypervascular lesions with numerous multinucleated giant cells.

29. **The answer is K.** Leukoplakia (Greek, "white plaque") is a descriptive term for many reactive, preneoplastic, and neoplastic lesions of the oral mucosa. *Squamous cell carcinoma* is found in a small minority (<10%) of such lesions.

30. **The answer is K.** *Squamous cell carcinoma* is the most common malignant tumor of the mouth. Carcinogenic factors that lead to the induction of cancer usually affect more than one site in the oral mucosa, and the tumors may therefore be multiple. Multiple tumors may develop at the same time (synchronous) or sequentially (metachronous).

31. **The answer is E.** Endemic *Burkitt lymphoma* occurs in African children and often presents as an extranodal lymphoma that involves the jaws.

32. **The answer is J.** *Pleomorphic adenoma* (mixed tumor) is the most common tumor of the major salivary glands, accounting for approximately two-thirds of all neoplasms. It occurs most commonly in the parotid.

Chapter 26

Bones and Joints

Questions

DIRECTIONS: Match each numbered statement with the most appropriate lettered item. Each lettered item can be used once, more than once, or not at all.

Bone and Joint Diseases

A. Achondroplasia
B. Ankylosing spondylitis
C. Avascular osteonecrosis
D. Chondrocalcinosis (pseudogout)
E. Infectious arthritis
F. Gout
G. Osteopetrosis
H. Osteitis cystica fibrosa (von Recklinghausen disease)
I. Osteoarthritis
J. Osteogenesis imperfecta
K. Osteomalacia
L. Osteomyelitis
M. Osteopetrosis
N. Paget disease
O. Reiter syndrome
P. Rheumatoid arthritis
Q. Still disease (juvenile arthritis)

_____ 1. A 30-year-old man suffered from congenital, inherited dwarfism and was admitted to the hospital for hip replacement due to severe osteoarthritis. He had short arms and legs and a relatively large head. Molecular biologic studies disclosed a mutation in the gene encoding the fibroblast growth factor receptor.

_____ 2. A 3-year-old boy had blue sclerae, was hard of hearing, and was treated for recurrent fractures of the long bones. He also had loose joints and abnormal teeth. Genetic testing demonstrated a mutation in the gene encoding pro-α1 collagen.

_____ 3. A 6-year-old child died of chronic infection and intractable chronic anemia. His bones were dense and misshapen. Histologically, they were composed of disorganized thick trabeculae, each of which contained a central core of calcified cartilage. Hemopoietic bone marrow cells were sparse.

_____ 4. A 10-year-old boy began limping shortly after a school soccer match and complained of increasing pain in his left hip. X-ray examination of the head of the femur showed a fracture and irregular densities of the cancellous bone. The parents were told that the boy had Legg-Calvé-Perthes disease.

_____ 5. A 9-year-old boy with fever of 2 weeks duration complained of pain and swelling in his left leg. X-ray examination revealed a lytic lesion surrounded by a sclerotic rim in the upper metaphysis of the tibia. A fine-needle aspiration demonstrated numerous neutrophils and cocci, and *Staphylococcus aureus* was cultured from the bone lesion.

_____ 6. A 50-year-old man complained of fever and severe pain in his great toe. The pain developed in the morning following his daughter's wedding and became so severe that he could not walk. Laboratory findings included leukocytosis, hyperuricemia, and hyperlipidemia. X-ray of the affected joint revealed lytic ("rat-bite"), punched-out lesions in the juxta-articular bone.

_____ 7. A 40-year-old woman complained of morning stiffness in her hands, and her finger joints were painful, swollen, and warm. X-ray examination showed narrowing of the joint spaces and erosion of joint surfaces of the metacarpal/phalangeal joints. The adjacent bones showed osteoporosis. She responded well to nonsteroidal anti-inflammatory drugs.

_____ 8. Sacroileitis and typical "bamboo-spine" were diagnosed radiologically in a 40-year-old man. He started noticing morning stiffness in his lower back during his college years. Lately, this stiffness had been accompanied by dull pain that during the past few weeks would wake him at night. He also noticed occasional pain in his right eye, accompanied by sensitivity to light. Rheumatoid factor and ANA were negative. The patient had the HLA-B27 major histocompatibility complex allele.

_____ 9. A 28-year-old man had a 3-day episode of diarrhea that subsided without treatment. However, he experienced burning pain on urination, and pain in his fingers and left eye. All the laboratory findings were within normal limits, except for mild anemia. He responded well to treatment with indomethacin.

_____ 10. A 10-year-old girl was examined by her family physician because of chronic pain in her hand and foot joints. She had no systemic symptoms. All the serologic and routine laboratory findings were normal.

_____ 11. An 85-year-old man noticed a painful swelling of his right knee. Joint fluid was aspirated and was found to contain numerous neutrophils and crystals, which were described as rhomboid and "coffinlike." Chemical analysis showed that they were composed of calcium pyrophosphate.

DIRECTIONS: Choose the one best answer.

_____ 12. Vertebral osteoblastic metastases of breast cancer are characterized by an elevation of serum
   A. acid phosphatase.
   B. alkaline phosphatase.
   C. alpha-1-antitrypsin.
   D. amylase.
   E. α-fetoprotein.

_____ 13. Which of the following diseases may cause numerous intrauterine fractures?
   A. Achondroplasia
   B. Osteoporosis
   C. Osteopetrosis
   D. Osteogenesis imperfecta
   E. Scurvy

_____ 14. Aseptic necrosis of bones is a well-known complication of all the following *except*
   A. air embolism in caisson disease.
   B. sickle cell anemia.
   C. polycythemia vera.
   D. corticosteroid administration.
   E. osteomyelitis.

_____ 15. Amyloidosis is a complication of
   A. osteoporosis.
   B. chronic osteomyelitis.
   C. avascular bone necrosis.
   D. renal osteodystrophy.
   E. enchondromatosis.

_____ 16. Reduced mineralization of osteoid is the underlying defect in
   A. osteoporosis.
   B. osteomalacia.
   C. osteonecrosis.
   D. osteopetrosis.
   E. myositis ossificans.

_____ 17. Osteopenia due to osteoporosis or osteomalacia is a complication of all the following *except*
   A. Cushing syndrome.
   B. virilizing adrenal tumor.
   C. primary biliary cirrhosis.
   D. intestinal malabsorption syndromes.
   E. multiple myeloma.

_____ 18. A fracture of the head of the humerus in an 80-year-old woman, which is associated with radiologically diagnosed osteopenia, is most likely caused by
   A. osteomalacia.
   B. osteoporosis.
   C. osteogenesis imperfecta.
   D. osteopetrosis.
   E. achondroplasia.

_____ **19.** All the following statements about osteoporosis are true *except*
A. it may cause enlargement of parathyroid glands.
B. it is associated with normal levels of calcium and phosphate in blood.
C. in bone biopsies, bone trabeculae appear fewer and thinner than normal but are normally calcified.
D. it is more common in women.
E. its highest prevalence is among the elderly.

_____ **20.** Renal osteodystrophy is primarily caused by
A. retention of calcium.
B. retention of phosphate.
C. calciuria.
D. reduced secretion of parathyroid hormone.
E. excess vitamin D in the circulation.

_____ **21.** A lytic lesion of the jaw, in an adult patient, which is histologically composed of osteoclasts and accompanied by hypercalcemia suggests the diagnosis of
A. end-stage kidney disease.
B. primary hyperparathyroidism.
C. rickets.
D. multiple myeloma.
E. giant cell tumor of bone.

_____ **22.** All the following are true of Paget disease *except*
A. it affects elderly individuals.
B. it may be mono-ostotic or polyostotic.
C. there is an imbalance between osteoblastic and osteoclastic activity.
D. it may undergo sarcomatous change.
E. deformed long bones result from cortical bone thinning.

_____ **23.** All the following are true of osteogenic sarcoma *except*
A. overall, it is the most common tumor within bone.
B. the peak incidence occurs between 10 and 20 years of age.
C. it is most often found in long bones around the knee.
D. osteoid and woven bone occur in the tumor.
E. metastases to the lungs are common.

_____ **24.** Which of the following is true for chondrosarcoma?
A. The peak incidence is between 10 and 20 years.
B. It usually presents as a juxtacortical lesion.
C. The short bones of the extremities are the most common site.
D. It usually originates from the epiphyseal growth plate.
E. A slow growth rate is typical.

_____ **25.** A 16-year-old boy presented with a tumor of the tibia. The x-ray showed a neoplasm permeating the diaphysis and subperiostal new bone formation in an "onion skin pattern." Histologically, the tumor was composed of "small blue cells." This tumor is a
A. form of lymphoma.
B. Ewing sarcoma.
C. osteogenic sarcoma.
D. chondrosarcoma of bone.
E. giant cell tumor.

_____ **26.** All the following are true of osteoarthritis *except*
   A. it is the most common form of joint disease in the United States.
   B. the incidence increases with the age of population.
   C. there is loss of articular cartilage.
   D. subchondral bone appears thickened radiologically.
   E. the metacarpal/phalangeal joints are first involved.

_____ **27.** All the following characterize rheumatoid arthritis *except*
   A. it is a systemic disease.
   B. the serologic findings are diagnostic.
   C. chronic synovitis with pannus formation occurs.
   D. there is juxtaarticular bone loss.
   E. subcutaneous granulomas with central areas of fibrinoid necrosis occur.

_____ **28.** Which of the following statements is true of gout?
   A. It is more often secondary to another condition than it is primary (i.e., idiopathic).
   B. Clinical symptoms occur in all those who have hyperuricemia.
   C. The joints of the great toes are the most common site of gouty arthritis.
   D. Females are more often affected than males.
   E. A tophus usually occurs centrally (i.e., in the heart or lungs).

_____ **29.** All the following are true of soft-tissue tumors *except*
   A. the more superficial the location, the more likely the tumor is to be benign.
   B. the larger the tumor, the more likely it is to be malignant.
   C. rapidly growing tumors are more likely to be malignant.
   D. benign tumors are more vascular by angiography than malignant ones.
   E. calcifications in the tumor have no prognostic implications.

_____ **30.** Which of the following soft-tissue lesions has a biphasic histologic pattern and consists of cuboidal epithelial and spindle-shaped mesenchymal cells?
   A. Nodular fasciitis
   B. Malignant fibrous histiocytoma
   C. Liposarcoma
   D. Rhabdomyosarcoma
   E. Synovial sarcoma

A n s w e r s

1. **The answer is A.** *Achondroplasia* is the most common inherited form of dwarfism and represents an autosomal dominant trait. It results from the mutation of the FGF receptor. This genetic defect leads to abnormal endochondral ossification, which impedes the growth of long bones of the extremities. The calvaria develop normally; thus the head appears relatively large in comparison with the extremities.

2. **The answer is J.** *Osteogenesis imperfecta* includes several congenital disorders caused by mutations of genes encoding the proteins that form the collagen type I triple helix. This child most likely has type I osteogenesis imperfecta. Abnormal collagen accounts for blue sclerae, skeletal fragility, deafness, laxity of joints, and dental abnormalities.

3. **The answer is M.** *Osteopetrosis* (also known as marble bone disease) is an autosomal recessive disorder characterized by abnormally dense bones. The condition is presumably related to hypofunction of osteoclasts. Abnormal bone trabeculae, which contain a central cartilaginous core, compress the bone marrow, causing anemia and bone marrow failure.

4. **The answer is C.** *Avascular osteonecrosis* (also known as aseptic necrosis) is a term used to describe bone infarcts caused by a variety of conditions, such as trauma, thrombi, emboli, corticosteroids, and so on. Growing bones of children and adolescents are often affected, and in most instances the cause of such infarctions is not evident. Legg-Calvé-Perthes disease is the eponym for avascular necrosis of the head of the femur.

5. **The answer is K.** *Osteomyelitis* caused by pyogenic bacteria produces lytic lesions of the bone, typically associated with fever, leukocytosis, and systemic signs of infection. Primary bone infection occurs most often in the metaphysis of long bones of growing children and adolescents. *Staphylococcus aureus* accounts for 80% to 90% of all cases.

6. **The answer is F.** *Gout* is a heterogeneous group of diseases characterized by hyperuricemia and the deposition of uric acid crystals in tissues. Joints (especially the metatarsal/phalangeal joint of the great toe) are often affected. Crystals of uric acid attract neutrophils, causing acute inflammation. Chronic accumulation of uric acid crystals leads to the formation of nodules (tophi) that contain granulomalike aggregates of macrophages. Acute episodes of gout often follow gluttonous intake of alcohol and food, and in this case could have been precipitated by the wedding party.

7. **The answer is Q.** *Rheumatoid arthritis* is a chronic systemic disease affecting preferentially small joints, most often the metacarpal/phalangeal joints at the hand. Rheumatoid factor is present in 80% of cases, and other signs of altered cellular immunity indicate that the disease is immune-mediated. The inflammation in the joints leads to the formation of pannus (granulation tissue covering the joint surface), resulting in typical x-ray findings.

8. **The answer is B.** *Ankylosing spondylitis* is an HLA-B27-linked inflammatory disease that usually involves the sacroiliac joints. The disease is progressive and leads to ossification of spinal joints, recognizable radiologically as a "bamboo-spine."

9. **The answer is O.** *Reiter syndrome* is a triad comprising arthritis, conjunctivitis, and urethritis. It occurs almost exclusively in man. Of those with this syndrome, 90% have the HLA-B27 haplotype. Attacks are often precipitated by infection such as dysentery or a sexually transmitted disease.

10. **The answer is Q.** *Still disease* (juvenile arthritis) is a term for a variety of joint diseases in children. About a fourth of all cases are "seronegative" and have no systemic symptoms.

11. **The answer is D.** *Chondrocalcinosis* (pseudogout) is an old-age disease that is characterized by deposits of calcium pyrophosphate. Chalky white layers on the joint surfaces are noted.

12. **The answer is B.** Osteoblasts express *alkaline phosphatase* on their plasma membranes. This enzyme is released into the blood in increased amounts in conditions marked by osteoblastic proliferation, such as callus formation or osteoblastic metastases. Osteoblasts may also be present in osteolytic bone lesions, but little, if any, of their lysosomal acid phosphatase enters the blood. Alpha-1-antitrypsin, amylase, and α-feto-protein are not secreted by bone cells.

13. **The answer is D.** *Osteogenesis imperfecta* causes fragility of bones and leads to multiple fractures, which, in severe cases of the disease, may even occur in utero. In achondroplasia fractures of deformed bones may occur in later life, but are not found in utero. Although bones in osteopetrosis are less resistant to stress than normal bones, intrauterine fractures do not occur.

    Scurvy, a disease caused by vitamin C deficiency, is marked by insufficient formation of collagen by osteoblasts, which results in inadequate formation of woven bone, disorganized epiphyseal plates, and abnormally soft bones. Scurvy could theoretically affect the fetus in utero, but that occurs very rarely, if ever.

14. **The answer is E.** *Aseptic necrosis of bone* occurs in many conditions in which the blood supply to the bone is compromised (e.g., sickle cell anemia and hyperviscosity syndromes, such as polycythemia vera or air embolism of caisson disease). However, in most cases, the cause is obscure. Foci of bone necrosis occur in osteomyelitis, but these should be considered "septic" rather than aseptic.

15. **The answer is B.** Amyloidosis is a complication of many chronic suppurative diseases, including *osteomyelitis*. Chronic osteomyelitis and tuberculosis of bones were previously common causes of amyloidosis but are rare today.

16. **The answer is B.** *Osteomalacia* is characterized by impaired mineralization of the osteoid. It is principally caused by a deficiency of vitamin D or its abnormal metabolism. Osteomalacia differs from osteoporosis, which is an imbalance between bone formation and resorption that results in a net loss of bone. In osteomalacia the bony trabeculae are rimmed by broad layers of osteoid, whereas the bone spicules in osteoporosis are thin but normally mineralized.

17. **The answer is B.** Because *androgens stimulate bone formation*, androgen-producing (virilizing) *adrenal tumors* would not be expected to produce osteoporosis. Corticosteroids are probably the most common cause of osteoporosis. In primary biliary cirrhosis and intestinal malabsorption syndromes, for example, sprue develops because defective absorption of vitamin D causes osteoporosis or osteomalacia. Multiple myeloma is a tumor of the bone marrow that causes osteoporosis by promoting bone resorption.

18. **The answer is B.** Osteopenia and fractures of long bones in elderly women are most often caused by *osteoporosis.*

19. **The answer is A.** Osteoporosis does not affect the homeostasis of calcium and phosphate. Blood levels of calcium and phosphate are normal; there is no hyperparathyroidism, and the parathyroid glands are of normal size.

20. **The answer is B.** Renal osteodystrophy, a feature of chronic renal disease, is primarily caused by *renal retention of phosphate.* Phosphate levels in the serum are elevated, and calcium is either normal or low. By contrast, primary hyperparathyroidism is marked by hypercalcemia and low serum phosphate levels. There is an increased secretion of parathyroid hormone in both conditions. In renal osteodystrophy it is compensatory for low serum calcium, whereas in primary hyperparathyroidism it reflects autonomous hyperfunction or a tumor of the parathyroid glands. In both cases, the parathyroid glands are enlarged, and the stimulatory effects of parathyroid hormone on osteoclasts enhance the resorption of bones.

21. **The answer is B.** Aggregates of osteoclasts in lytic bone lesions are known as "brown tumors." They are features of *primary hyperparathyroidism* and do not occur in renal osteodystrophy, rickets, or multiple myeloma. Brown tumors of hyperparathyroidism do not differ histologically from primary giant cell tumors of bones, but only the former is associated with hypercalcemia.

22. **The answer is E.** Paget disease is a disorder of unknown origin, which occurs in older people and involves either a single bone or several bones. It is not associated with systemic metabolic disturbances, and some parts of the skeleton are always spared. The bones show *marked thickening,* owing to excessive osteoblastic and reduced osteoclastic activity. Although only few persons suffering from Paget disease develop sarcoma of bone, in adults the disease remains an important predisposing condition for this tumor in long bones. The skull and vertebrae are virtually never the site of secondary osteogenic sarcomas.

23. **The answer is A.** Osteosarcoma is the most common primary malignant tumor of bones. However, primary malignant tumors of bones are rare, and *metastases from other primary sites to the bones are far more common.* Osteogenic sarcomas typically arise in young people, with a peak incidence between 10 and 20 years of age. They originate preferentially in the metaphyses of growing long bones; the lower end of the femur and the upper ends of the tibia and fibula are the most common sites. Histologically, the tumor is composed of malignant osteoblasts, which may (a) produce only collagen type I and thus be indistinguishable from fibroblasts; (b) form recognizable osteoid; or (c) produce spicules of woven bone. The tumor metastasizes hematogenously and tends to spread to the lungs early in the course of the disease.

24. **The answer is E.** Chondrosarcoma originates from remnants of cartilage within bones and most often involves the deeper portions of the pelvic bones of middle-aged or older people. It may arise in long bones, but the short bones of the hand and foot are rarely involved. The tumor is composed of malignant cartilage cells showing different degrees of maturation. Chondrosarcomas usually *grow slowly.*

25. **The answer is B.** Ewing sarcoma is a *diaphysial tumor* that on x-ray shows an "onion skin" pattern, owing to the layers of newly formed reactive bone in the periosteum. Although the tumor is composed of small, basophilic cells that resemble lymphocytes, it is not a lymphoma. The tumor tends to metastasize to other bones and to other internal organs.

26. **The answer is E.** Osteoarthritis, or degenerative joint disease, is the most common disease of the joints. This "wear-and-tear" disorder affects the articular cartilage, which is slowly destroyed. The underlying bone is thus exposed to increased stress. Thickening (apparent by x-ray) and restructuring of the subchondral bone produce the appearance of ivory ("eburnization"). Weight-carrying joints are commonly affected. The *metacarpal/phalangeal joints* are distorted in rheumatoid arthritis.

27. **The answer is B.** Rheumatoid arthritis is a systemic disease in which immune mechanisms play a crucial role. The disorder is associated with serologic findings, such as rheumatoid factor and various autoantibodies. However, *none of these autoantibodies is pathognomonic*, and many may be found in asymptomatic older persons. Joint inflammation is invariably present. The formation of a pannus and a hyperplastic synovium infiltrated with lymphocytes and other chronic inflammatory cells are characteristic. The pannus may lead to ankylosis (i.e., immobilization of the obliterated joint). The bone surrounding the immobile joint undergoes rarefaction and localized osteoporosis. Rheumatoid nodules occur most often in subcutaneous regions at pressure points. They are composed of granulomas, with central aggregates of fibrin, immunoglobulin, and serum proteins, which are traditionally called *fibrinoid*.

28. **The answer is C.** Gout presents with swelling and pain in the first *metatarsal/phalangeal joints of the big toe* in at least 50% of patients. The older term *podagra* (Greek, "trap for the foot") attests to the prevalence of this presentation. Gout is in most instances idiopathic (i.e., the cause of hyperuricemia is unknown). Typically, it affects males (95%), with a peak incidence in the fifth decade. Tophi (i.e., nodular deposits of monosodium urate crystals) occur in the cartilage, connective tissue of the joints, and subcutaneous tissues of the extremities.

29. **The answer is D.** *Malignant tumors tend to elicit a stronger angiogenic response than benign ones.*

30. **The answer is E.** *Synovial cell sarcoma* often consists of spindle-shaped mesenchymal cells and cuboidal epitheliallike cells. The latter stain with antibodies to keratin, form glands and clefts, and are presumably epithelial. All the other tumors listed exhibit some histologic polymorphism, but their cells do not show any epithelial features or markers of differentiation.

Chapter 27

Skeletal Muscle

Questions

DIRECTIONS: Match each numbered statement with the most appropriate lettered item. Each lettered item can be used once, more than once, or not at all.

Diseases of Muscles

      A. Becker muscular dystrophy
      B. Carnitine palmityl transferase deficiency
      C. Dermatomyositis
      D. Duchenne muscular dystrophy
      E. Facioscapulohumeral muscular dystrophy
      F. Lambert-Eaton myasthenic syndrome
      G. Limb-girdle muscular dystrophy
      H. Myasthenia gravis
      I. Myotonic dystrophy
      J. Oculopharyngeal muscular dystrophy
      K. Polymyositis
      L. Toxic myopathy

_____ 1. A muscle biopsy was performed on the calf muscle of a 16-year-old boy who experienced easy fatigability and muscle weakness. The muscle showed marked variation in size and shape of muscle fibers. There were foci of muscle fiber necrosis, with myophagocytosis, regenerating fibers and fibrosis. A patchy distribution of dystrophin was demonstrated immunohisto-chemically, and the intensity of the staining was weaker than that in the normal control muscle.

_____ 2. A 10-year-old girl complained of persistent redness of the skin over her knuckles and around the nailbeds. The upper eyelids had a lilac discoloration. She noted easy fatigability and could rise only with difficulty from a squatting position. Creatine kinase was elevated in the blood. A muscle biopsy revealed infiltrates of lymphocytes and macrophages surrounding dead and dying muscle fibers, and perifascicular atrophy of muscle fibers.

_____ **3.** A 60-year-old man who had been treated for stomach cancer complained of a rash on his chest and pain in his upper arms and calves. He could not raise his arms and climbed the stairs only with difficulty. A muscle biopsy revealed perivascular infiltrates of lymphocytes and plasma cells extending in between the muscle fibers.

_____ **4.** A 4-year-old boy tended to fall easily, could not jump, and would easily tire during exercise. The neurologist documented pronounced muscle weakness in all four extremities. Creatine kinase was elevated in the blood, and electromyography showed myopathic changes. A muscle biopsy showed pronounced muscle fiber necrosis and regeneration. Myophagocytosis and intramysial fibrosis were prominent. Dystrophin was absent from all muscle fibers by immunohistochemical staining.

_____ **5.** A 20-year-old woman complained of fatigability and muscle weakness, most prominently in the shoulders and upper arms. Her sister and brother had similar problems. Her face was tense and expressionless. A neurologic examination revealed "winging scapulae," sloping shoulders, and weakness of trapezius, biceps, and triceps muscles. Creatine kinase levels in the blood were only slightly elevated. Electromyography suggested myopathic changes. A muscle biopsy revealed mild nondiagnostic alterations, such as focal muscle fiber atrophy, compensatory hypertrophy, and scattered "moth-eaten" fibers, best demonstrated by enzyme histochemistry.

_____ **6.** A 25-year-old woman noticed weakness and easy fatigability, most pronounced in the late afternoon. She experienced difficulty in reading and tiredness while watching television. She had problems chewing and swallowing and lost her voice while talking. Her condition improved after the thymectomy.

_____ **7.** A 70-year-old man who had been treated for small cell carcinoma of the lung developed marked weakness of his legs and arms. He also complained of mouth dryness, double vision, and a drooping upper eyelid. EMG showed incremental responses to stimulation. Antibodies against the calcium channel of the nerve terminals were found in the blood. A muscle biopsy was normal.

_____ **8.** A 40-year-old man was referred to a neurologist for evaluation of muscle weakness. He had marked atrophy of leg and arm muscles, fixed facial expression, and pronounced temporal baldness. He could not open his hand for a handshake and could not extend his arm after flexing it. He was found to have testicular atrophy and diabetes. A muscle biopsy revealed atrophy of type I fibers, ring fibers, and numerous fibers with centrally located nuclei.

_____ **9.** A 20-year-old man had experienced pronounced bouts of muscle cramps following jogging and had noticed darkening of his urine. Although a muscle biopsy displayed no morphologic abnormalities, a deficiency of an enzyme involved in lipid metabolism was demonstrated biochemically.

_____ **10.** The presence of scattered, small, angulated muscle fibers was noticed in a muscle biopsy of a 60-year-old diabetic man with distal muscle weakness. What is the most likely diagnosis?
A. Becker muscular dystrophy
B. Dermatomyositis
C. Myotonic dystrophy
D. Neurogenic muscle atrophy
E. Polymyositis

_____ **11.** Variation in size and shape of muscle fibers, combined with degenerative changes and intramysial fibrosis, is typical of
A. denervation atrophy.
B. denervation of muscle with reinnervation.
C. muscular dystrophy.
D. mitochondrial myopathy.
E. myasthenia gravis.

_____ **12.** Progressive muscular dystrophy of Duchenne is characterized by all the following *except*
A. elevated levels of creatine kinase are detectable in utero.
B. muscle weakness occurs initially in the shoulder/pelvic girdle.
C. patients are usually confined to a wheelchair by the age of 10 years.
D. death is due to respiratory insufficiency.
E. boys and girls are affected equally.

_____ **13.** In a female child born with severe hypotonia of skeletal muscles, all the following should be considered *except*
A. Werdnig-Hoffman disease.
B. glycogenosis.
C. nonprogressive lower motor neuron disease.
D. congenital myopathy.
E. periodic paralysis.

_____ **14.** Elevated levels of serum creatine kinase (CK) are found in all the following *except*
A. polymyositis.
B. rhabdomyolysis.
C. myositis of systemic lupus erythematosus.
D. muscular dystrophy.
E. myasthenia gravis.

_____ **15.** Dermatomyositis of middle-aged or older men is commonly associated with
A. coronary artery disease.
B. cancer.
C. cirrhosis of the liver.
D. emphysema.
E. Alzheimer disease.

_____ 16. The presence of eosinophils in a muscle biopsy is most consistent with a diagnosis of
A. autoimmune polymyositis.
B. bacterial myositis.
C. myositis due to coxsackie virus infection.
D. *Trichinella spiralis* infection.
E. *Treponema pallidum* infection.

_____ 17. Which of the following is characterized by denervation atrophy of the muscles?
A. Carnitine palmityl transferase deficiency
B. McArdle disease
C. Pompe disease
D. Werdnig-Hoffman disease
E. Myoadenylate deaminase deficiency

_____ 18. Selective type II muscle fiber atrophy occurs in all the following conditions *except*
A. disuse atrophy.
B. cerebral palsy.
C. cerebral apoplexy.
D. steroid therapy.
E. amyotrophic lateral sclerosis.

_____ 19. Myasthenia gravis is most often associated with tumors of the
A. brain.
B. lung.
C. thymus.
D. liver.
E. kidney.

_____ 20. In myasthenia gravis the neuromuscular junctions contain deposits of
A. acetylcholine.
B. acetylcholine receptor antigens.
C. acetylcholinesterase.
D. immunoglobulin.
E. myoglobin.

A n s w e r s

1. **The answer is A.** *Becker muscular dystrophy* is an X-linked recessive disorder caused by mutations in the dystrophin gene and can be considered a mild form of Duchenne dystrophy. Symptoms of muscle weakness usually appear in adolescence. Dystrophin is abnormal but may be demonstrated immunohistochemically in the muscle fiber, albeit in a patchy distribution.

2. **The answer is C.** *Dermatomyositis* often affects girls and young women, presenting with skin changes and muscle symptoms. The proximal muscles are preferentially involved. Muscle inflammation is best demonstrated by biopsy. CK released from injured muscle fibers contributes to high levels of the enzyme in the blood.

3. **The answer is C.** *Dermatomyositis* in the elderly is often a paraneoplastic syndrome. Histologic signs of muscle inflammation are diagnostic.

4. **The answer is D.** *Duchenne muscular dystrophy* is an X-linked recessive disorder related to mutations of the gene encoding dystrophin. Signs of muscle weakness and wasting occur early in childhood. Damaged muscle fibers release CK into the blood. Accordingly, CK levels are elevated in all patients. Damaged muscle fibers are removed by macrophages and replaced by fibrous tissue and fat (pseudohypertrophy).

5. **The answer is E.** *Facioscapulohumeral muscular dystrophy* is a mild disorder that presents clinically in the 20- to 40-year age group. It is an autosomal dominant muscle disease that affects the muscles of the face, upper torso, and upper arms. Changes in the muscle biopsy are mild and nondiagnostic.

6. **The answer is H.** *Myasthenia gravis* is an autoimmune disorder characterized by the deposition of antibodies to acetylcholine receptors at the neuromuscular junction. These antibodies inhibit the transmission of nerve impulses but produce no pathologic changes. Hence a muscle biopsy is not indicated, and the diagnosis is made on the basis of typical clinical findings indicative of muscle weakness. EMG shows a myasthenic pattern (loss of responsiveness to repeat stimuli) and a good response to cholinesterase inhibitors (e.g., edrophonium), which improves muscle contraction. When myasthenia of young women is associated with thymoma or thymic hyperplasia, it responds well to thymectomy.

7. **The answer is F.** *Lambert-Eaton myasthenic syndrome* is a paraneoplastic condition that presents as a myasthenia-like muscle weakness. Most patients have small cell carcinoma of the lung. They develop antibodies to calcium channels in the nerve endings at the neuromuscular junction, which inhibit the transmission of neural impulses. In contrast to myasthenia gravis, electrical stimulation creates an incremental response. Autonomic symptoms such as mouth dryness and impotence are often present.

8. **The answer is I.** *Myotonic dystrophy* is an autosomal dominant disorder related to a triple nucleotide repeat on chromosome 19. Muscle weakness appears in adult life and is typically associated with myotonia and endocrine disorders, such as diabetes mellitus or testicular hypofunction. EMG shows typical spastic contractions upon stimulation and lack of relaxation.

9. **The answer is B.** *Carnitine palmityl transferase deficiency* is an inborn error of lipid metabolism that causes muscle weakness and cramps. Rhabdomyolysis during cramps may result in myoglobinuria, which presents with darkening of the urine. The muscle biopsy shows no significant morphologic changes, and the diagnosis rests on biochemical documentation of the enzyme deficiency.

10. **The answer is D.** *Denervation* of single muscle fibers results in altered size and shape. Compressed by the surrounding normal fibers, atrophic fibers are molded to the contours of adjacent fibers and thus appear angular.

11. **The answer is C.** Variation in the size and shape of muscle fibers, degenerative changes in some fibers, and intrafascicular fibrosis are features of

muscular dystrophy. Denervation presents with scattered atrophic fibers that assume an angulated shape; most other fibers appear normal. Reinnervation is characterized by type-specific grouping of fibers, which is assessed by enzyme histochemistry. Mitochondrial myopathy is diagnosed only by enzyme histochemistry or electron microscopy, which discloses abnormal mitochondria or an increased number of mitochondria. Myasthenia gravis shows either no histologic changes in the muscle or aggregates of lymphocytes in the muscle fibers.

12. **The answer is E.** Duchenne muscular dystrophy is an X-linked recessive disorder that is transmitted by unaffected female carriers and *affects males exclusively*. The disease causes muscle cell degeneration and necrosis, with a consequent elevation of muscle-derived creatine kinase (CK) in the blood. High levels of CK may also be found in the amniotic fluid. The disease begins early in life. By the age of 3 to 4 years, most boys show pelvic and shoulder girdle weakness. They are usually bound to a wheelchair by age 10. Progressive muscular disease finally involves the heart and respiratory muscles, and death is usually due to cardiorespiratory failure.

13. **The answer is E.** *Periodic paralysis* is associated with abnormalities in potassium metabolism and, unlike the other diseases listed, does not present at birth. Werdnig-Hoffman disease is a severe form of congenital hypotonia caused by the degeneration of anterior spinal cord neurons. Inborn errors of carbohydrate metabolism (e.g., Pompe disease [glycogenosis type II]) also cause hypotonia at birth and in early infancy. Congenital myopathies are a diverse group of muscle disorders that present with hypotonia and include entities such as central core disease, rod (nemaline) myopathy, and central nuclear myopathy.

14. **The answer is E.** Elevated levels of CK in the blood are found in all muscle disorders that are characterized by the destruction of muscle fibers. Since there is no muscle cell necrosis in *myasthenia gravis*, serum CK activity is not increased.

15. **The answer is B.** Dermatomyositis occurs primarily as an isolated autoimmune disorder, mostly in girls and young women, or as part of a complex multisystem disease. When it occurs in older men, it is usually a paraneoplastic condition, most commonly in association with lung *cancer*.

16. **The answer is D.** Eosinophils in the muscle are commonly found in association with parasitic infections, the most common being *trichinosis*. Autoimmune polymyositis is characterized by infiltrates of lymphocytes and macrophages. Bacterial infections elicit a polymorphonuclear reaction, and syphilis is marked by infiltrates of lymphocytes and plasma cells around small blood vessels.

17. **The answer is D.** *Werdnig-Hoffman disease* is an autosomal recessive, congenital, muscular hypotonia characterized by marked neurogenic muscular atrophy. This condition is also called "infantile spinal muscular atrophy" and is primarily due to the destruction of the anterior horn cells in the spinal cord. All other diseases listed are metabolic myopathies, representing inborn errors of carbohydrate metabolism (McArdle and Pompe disease), lipid metabolism (carnitine palmityl transferase deficiency), and purine metabolism (myoadenylate deaminase deficiency).

18. **The answer is E.** *Amyotrophic lateral sclerosis* is a motor neuron disease, and atrophy of muscle is characterized by nonselective shrinkage of both type I and type II fibers. By contrast, upper motor neuron injury, such as occurs in cerebral palsy or following a stroke, is similar to disuse atrophy in being marked by selective atrophy of type II fibers. So-called steroid myopathy also presents as type II muscle cell atrophy.

19. **The answer is C.** *Thymic abnormalities* are found in more than two-thirds of patients with myasthenia gravis. Most show only follicular hyperplasia of the thymus, but 10% to 15% have a thymoma. By contrast, 50% to 60% of all patients with thymoma have symptoms of myasthenia gravis.

20. **The answer is D.** Antibodies to the acetylcholine receptor can be demonstrated in the serum of most patients with myasthenia gravis. These *immunoglobulins* are deposited at the neuromuscular junction and can be demonstrated immunohistochemically in muscle biopsies.

Chapter 28

Nervous System

Questions

DIRECTIONS: Match each numbered statement with the most appropriate lettered item. Each lettered item can be used once, more than once, or not at all.

Diseases of the Central Nervous System

    A. AIDS-related encephalopathy
    B. Alzheimer disease
    C. Amyotrophic lateral sclerosis
    D. Creutzfeldt-Jakob disease
    E. Hepatic encephalopathy
    F. Huntington disease
    G. Metachromatic leukodystrophy
    H. Multiple sclerosis
    I. Parkinson disease
    J. Poliomyelitis
    K. Progressive multifocal leukoencephalopathy
    L. Rabies
    M. Stroke (cerebrovascular accident)
    N. Tabes dorsalis
    O. Vitamin B_{12} deficiency
    P. Wernicke encephalopathy

_____ **1.** A 45-year-old man who was known to have a syphilitic aneurysm of the thoracic aorta developed a "staggering" gait and lightning pain in his hands and legs. The neurologic examination revealed impaired senses of vibration, touch, and pain in all extremities. He contracted pneumonia and died. The autopsy disclosed selective loss of axons in the posterior columns of the spinal cord.

_____ **2.** A 75-year-old man was increasingly becoming forgetful and withdrawn. The patient's mental condition progressively deteriorated and he died 10 years later. At autopsy the brain showed marked narrowing of the gyri, widening of the sulci, and dilatation of the lateral ventricles. Histologically, it demonstrated neurofibrillary tangles, granulovacuolar degeneration, neuritic plaques, and deposits of amyloid.

_____ **3.** The wife of a 50-year-old man noticed that after a major automobile accident he had become withdrawn, did not talk, and had strange mood swings. He had to be hospitalized and died 6 month later. A spongiform encephalopathy was diagnosed at autopsy.

_____ **4.** A 35-year-old woman had several episodes of urinary incontinence, experienced pain in her left eye, and had visual difficulties. Funduscopic examination showed no abnormalities. Two months later she complained of double vision and numbness in the fingers of her left hand. A MRI showed multiple scattered lesions in the brain and spinal cord. On lumbar puncture, the CSF contained increased amounts of IgG. The patient's condition initially improved, but she had severe relapses and finally died 15 years after the onset of her first symptoms. The autopsy disclosed numerous plaques of demyelinated white matter.

_____ **5.** A 60-year-old man walked slowly and appeared stiff and stooped. He had an expressionless face and spoke in a monotonous voice. A tremor of the fingers was apparent, but it ceased when he tried to reach something. He died at the age of 80 years. At autopsy, the substantia nigra appeared pale, and numerous Lewy bodies were seen in that location.

_____ **6.** A 60-year-old chronic alcoholic was found in a state of mental confusion. The following neurologic symptoms were recorded: horizontal diplopia, strabismus, amblyopia, nystagmus, ataxia, and peripheral neuropathy. He died of pneumonia 2 days later. At autopsy the brain showed calcification and brownish discoloration of the atrophic mammillary bodies and periaqueductal regions of the midbrain and tegmentum of the pons.

_____ **7.** A 7-year-old boy died in a state of delirium 4 weeks after a trip to visit archeological caves. At autopsy the brain stem showed infiltrates of lymphocytes around small blood vessels. There was evidence of neuronophagia, and some neurons contained Negri bodies.

Intracranial Hemorrhages

    A. Cerebellar hemorrhage
    B. Epidural hematoma
    C. Intracerebral hemorrhage
    D. Intraventricular hemorrhage
    E. Pontine hemorrhage
    F. Subdural hematoma
    G. Subarachnoid hemorrhage

_____ **8.** This bleeding occurred following a fracture of the temporal-parietal bone. An initial asymptomatic period of a few hours was followed by rapid deterioration of brain functions and death within 24 hours.

_____ **9.** Bleeding from torn bridging veins in a boxer was attributed to repeated head trauma.

_____ **10.** Bleeding was traced to a ruptured saccular aneurysm of the circle of Willis (berry aneurysm).

Tumors of the Central Nervous System

A. Astrocytoma
B. Craniopharyngioma
C. Ependymoma
D. Ganglioglioma
E. Glioblastoma
F. Hemangioblastoma
G. Lymphoma
H. Medulloblastoma
I. Meningioma
J. Oligodendroglioma
K. Schwannoma

_____ **11.** Most common primary intracranial tumor
_____ **12.** Cystic tumor of the cerebellum in children
_____ **13.** Marked cellular pleomorphism and areas of necrosis
_____ **14.** Most commonly located in the fourth ventricle, but also found in the filum terminale
_____ **15.** Located exclusively in the cerebellum, with a peak incidence in the first decade of life
_____ **16.** Benign tumor that may be asymptomatic or cause seizures by compression
_____ **17.** A component of von Hippel-Lindau syndrome
_____ **18.** A complication of AIDS
_____ **19.** A feature of neurofibromatosis type II
_____ **20.** Suprasellar tumor originating from the remnants of Rathke pouch

DIRECTIONS: Choose the one best answer.

_____ **21.** Swollen neurons that contain numerous lysosomes filled with lipid are typical of
A. amyloidosis.
B. Huntington disease.
C. kuru.
D. Tay-Sachs disease.
E. multiple sclerosis.

_____ **22.** Wernicke syndrome is marked by
A. necrosis of white matter.
B. petechial hemorrhages in the mammillary bodies.
C. demyelination of the optic nerves.
D. loss of neurons from the frontal lobe cortex.
E. periventricular gliosis in the cerebral hemispheres.

_____ **23.** All the following apply to Parkinson disease *except*
    A. tremors at rest and muscular rigidity.
    B. involvement of dopaminergic neurons.
    C. primary involvement of the substantia nigra.
    D. secondary involvement of the parietal cortex.
    E. eosinophilic cytoplasmic inclusions.

_____ **24.** Which of the following statements about Huntington disease is true?
    A. Inherited as an recessive trait
    B. Causes bilateral atrophy of the cerebellum
    C. Commonly results in paranoid ideation and choreoathetosis
    D. Has clinical symptoms that begin early in childhood
    E. Is a prion disease

_____ **25.** Amyotrophic lateral sclerosis is marked by degeneration and loss of all the following *except*
    A. cerebellar Purkinje cells.
    B. anterior horn cells of the spinal cord.
    C. the lateral pyramidal pathway of the spinal cord.
    D. upper motor neurons in the cerebral cortex.
    E. motor nuclei of the brain stem.

_____ **26.** Isolated degeneration of the posterior columns of the spinal cord is found in
    A. tabes dorsalis.
    B. friedreich ataxia.
    C. vitamin B_{12} deficiency.
    D. amyotrophic lateral sclerosis.
    E. poliomyelitis.

_____ **27.** Alzheimer disease is characterized by all the following *except*
    A. granulovacuolar degeneration.
    B. amyloid deposits.
    C. neurofibrillary tangles.
    D. cortical atrophy.
    E. Lewy bodies.

_____ **28.** Dementia is a feature of all the following *except*
    A. Huntington disease.
    B. Alzheimer disease.
    C. Creutzfeldt-Jakob disease.
    D. Pick disease.
    E. multiple sclerosis.

_____ **29.** In distal axonopathy, presenting as "glove and stocking" neuropathy, the peripheral nerve shows all the following *except*
    A. breakdown of the myelin sheath.
    B. disintegration of the axon.
    C. Schwann cell reaction.
    D. karyolysis in motor neurons.
    E. axonal sprouting and regeneration.

_____ **30.** Which of of the following is the most common peripheral nerve disease caused by diabetes mellitus?
  A. Distal polyneuropathy
  B. Autonomic neuropathy
  C. Mononeuropathy
  D. Inflammatory neuropathy
  E. Paraproteinemic neuropathy

Answers

1. **The answer is N.** *Tabes dorsalis* is a feature of tertiary syphilis and is characterized by chronic fibrosing meningitis, which contricts the posterior root of the spinal cord. The posterior roots contain sensory nerves that originate in the spinal ganglia and form the posterior columns of the spinal cord. Compression of these sensory nerves causes lancinating pain in extremities. It also damages the transmission of proprioceptive impulses, causing gait disturbances (ataxia).

2. **The answer is B.** *Alzheimer disease* is the most common cause of dementia in the elderly. It is characterized by atrophy of the brain, which can be recognized by CT-scan as widening of the sulci, atrophy of the gyri, and widening of the lateral ventricles. Histologic findings distinguish Alzheimer disease from other causes of dementia (e.g., Pick disease or multiple strokes).

3. **The answer is D.** *Creutzfeldt-Jakob disease* is a fatal prion disease that causes spongiform encepholopathy and presents clinically as dementia of acute onset with a rapid downhill course. Many patients show movement abnormalities, such as myoclonus or gait disturbances, together with other motor or visual defects.

4. **The answer is H.** *Multiple sclerosis* is an immune-mediated demyelinating disease, which may present with a variety of symptoms, such as sensory deficits, sphincter weakness, and tremors. Forty percent of cases are marked by eye problems, such as loss of visual fields, blindness in one eye, or diplopia. In such cases the foci of demyelination are found in the optic nerve, but the disease may involve other parts of the brain as well. Plaques of demyelinated white matter are typically found around the lateral ventricles of the cerebrum, in the cerebellum, and in the spinal cord. The cerebrospinal fluid contains increased amounts of IgG, which can be separated electrophorectically into several "oligoclonal" bands.

5. **The answer is I.** *Parkinson disease* is a neurodegenerative disease of unknown etiology that presents with the symptoms described in the present patient. The brain shows loss of pigmentation in neurons in the substantia nigra and locus ceruleus. Many of the surrounding neurons contain cytoplasmic filamentous inclusions called Lewy bodies.

6. **The answer is P.** *Wernicke encephalopathy* results from vitamin B_1 (thiamine) deficiency. The disease is typically found in chronic alcoholics and presents with a set of ocular, cerebellar, and mental disturbances. Pathologic changes are typically found in the mammillary bodies and periaqueductal regions of the midbrain and the tegmentum of the brain. Atrophy of the superior portion of cerebellar vermis also occurs.

7. **The answer is L.** *Rabies* is a viral encephalitis transmitted in the saliva of wild and domestic carnivores (e.g., foxes, bats, dogs) and presents with convulsions, involuntary spasms, and delirium. The pathognomonic viral inclusions (Negri bodies) are found in the neurons of the brain stem, hippocampus, and Purkinje cells of the cerebellum.

8. **The answer is B.** An *epidural hematoma* usually results from a traumatic bone fracture that severs the middle meningeal artery. The blood, under arterial pressure, cleaves the dura from the bone and forms a space that expands slowly. There are usually no symptoms until the epidural hematoma reaches a volume of about 50 to 60 ml over a period of 6 to 10 hours. If untreated, the expanding hematoma compresses the brain and causes death in 1 to 2 days.

9. **The answer is F.** Head trauma tends to shear the *bridging veins* that cross the virtual space between the arachnoid and the internal surface of the dura (i.e., the subdural space). Owing to low pressure within the torn veins and external compression by the hematoma, *subdural hemorrhage* tends to stop spontaneously. The blood coagulates, and granulation tissue grows into it. Subdural bleeding occurs most often when the head strikes a fixed surface, in which case the hematomas are often bilateral. The organized subdural hematoma may enlarge because of repeated trauma, which causes rebleeding, or as a result of the osmotic effect of the decomposed blood.

10. **The answer is G.** *Subarachnoid bleeding* without involvement of the other compartments is rare and arises mostly from arteries located at the base of the brain. It can be caused by trauma or by spontaneous rupture of congenitally weak vessels at the circle of Willis ("berry aneurysms").

11. **The answer is E.** *Glioblastoma multiforme* is the most common (40%) primary malignant tumor in the cranial cavity. Metastases from other sites, however, are more common than primary brain malignancies.

12. **The answer is A.** *Astrocytomas* may be solid or cystic. In children they are typically cystic and located in the cerebellum.

13. **The answer is E.** *Glioblastoma multiforme* is a brain tumor composed of malignant astroglial cells that show marked pleomorphism and are often *multinucleated.* Owing to their invasive properties and vascular changes ("arteritic obliteration"), the tumors show patchy yellow areas of *necrosis* and red zones of *hemorrhage.* The term *multiforme* derives from the variegated gross appearance of these tumors and the histologic pleomorphism of the tumor cells. When the tumor invades the contralateral hemisphere across the corpus callosum, it presents as a *bilateral* "butterfly-like" lesion.

14. **The answer is C.** *Ependymomas* are benign tumors that originate from any surface covered by ependymal cells. They occur most often in the *fourth ventricle* but also originate from the lining of the *central canal* of the spinal cord and the filum terminale. Together with astrocytomas, ependymonas are the most common neoplasms of the spinal cord. Because of their central location, they cannot be easily resected.

15. **The answer is H.** *Medulloblastomas* originate exclusively in the cerebellum. Since they are close to the fourth ventricle, they may be disseminated by the circulating cerebrospinal fluid downstream into the spinal cord. Most medulloblastomas occur in children.

16. **The answer is I.** *Meningiomas* are biologically benign tumors of the arachnoid that tend to invade the overlying bone, a finding that helps in the radiologic identification of these tumors. Meningiomas grow slowly with an estimated doubling time of about 2 years. The tumors may be asymptomatic for years, and often the only symptoms are epileptic seizures caused by focal compression of the cerebral cortex.

17. **The answer is F.** *Hemangioblastomas* of the cerebellum are found in conjunction with retinal hemangiomas and are part of the hereditary von Hippel-Lindau syndrome.

18. **The answer is G.** *Lymphoma* of the brain is a well-known complication of AIDS.

19. **The answer is K.** *Schwannomas* of the auditory nerve are typical features of neurofibromatosis type II. They are usually bilateral.

20. **The answer is B.** *Craniopharyngioma* is a tumor derived from the epithelium of the Rathke pouch, a part of the embryonic nasopharynx that gives rise to the anterior lobe of the pituitary.

21. **The answer is D.** Swollen neurons that exhibit marked vacuolization of the perikaryon and contain lysosomes filled with lipid are found in *Tay-Sachs disease* but could occur in other *lipid-storage diseases* as well. The correct diagnosis can be established by biochemical analysis of the stored material or identification of intermediary metabolites and missing enzymes. The other diseases listed do not produce such neuronal changes.

22. **The answer is B.** *Wernicke syndrome* is caused by thiamine deficiency, usually in chronic alcoholics. It is marked clinically by an acute onset of altered consciousness, ophthalmoplegia, nystagmus, disturbances in thermoregulation, and ataxia. Histologic examination of the brain reveals petechiae in the mammillary bodies, hypothalamus, periaqueductal gray matter, and floor of the fourth ventricle.

23. **The answer is D.** *Parkinsonism* is a neurologic disease that involves the *substantia nigra and locus ceruleus.* Grossly visible depigmentation of these loci corresponds to a loss of dopaminergic neurons. Secondary changes occur in the striatum, the putamen being most prominently involved. The cerebral cortex is not affected. Clinically, the disease presents with tremor and muscular rigidity. Lewy bodies are a histologic hallmark of the disease.

24. **The answer is C.** *Huntington disease* is an *autosomal dominant disorder* that involves the *extrapyramidal system* and causes atrophy of both caudate nuclei. It reflects mutations of the HD gene on chromosome 4 and involves an expansion of an unstable trinucleotide (CAG) repeat. The *frontal cortex* undergoes symmetric atrophy. The most prominent extrapyramidal symptom is athetosis with chorea. The cortical lesions cause *mental changes,* paranoia, and delusions. During the first third to fifth decades of life the afflicted person remains asymptomatic.

25. **The answer is A.** *Amyotrophic lateral sclerosis* usually begins with degenerative changes in the *lateral pyramidal columns* in the lumbosacral spinal cord, although this pyramidal tract originates from upper motor neurons in the cerebral cortex. Other motor neurons in the spinal cord and in the brain stem progressively become involved, but the caudal/cepha-

lad gradient that is set at the onset of the disease persists. Purkinje cells in the cerebellum are not motor neurons and are unaffected.

26. **The answer is A.** *Tabes dorsalis* is marked by posterior column degeneration that results from compression atrophy of the posterior nerve roots caused by syphilitic meningitis and vasculitis. *Friedreich ataxia* is an autosomal dominant trait that involves the spinal cord in a complex way. It affects not only the centripetal pathways (spinocerebellar and posterior columns), but also the efferent corticospinal tracts. Subacute combined degeneration is due to vitamin B_{12} deficiency and involves not only the posterior columns, but also the anterior horn cells and the spinocerebellar and corticospinal tracts. Amyotrophic lateral sclerosis is a motor neuron disease that does not affect the posterior columns. Poliomyelitis involves anterior horn motor neurons.

27. **The answer is E.** Alzheimer disease shows prominent *granulovacuolar* degeneration of the cell cytoplasm of pyramidal cells in the hippocampus. *Neurofibrillary tangles* (i.e., aggregates of neurofilaments in the cytoplasm of neurons) are prominent and often associated with senile or *neuritic plaques* that contain amyloid. On gross examination, the disease is marked by widespread *cerebral cortical atrophy*. Lewy bodies occur in Parkinson disease.

28. **The answer is E.** *Huntington disease, Alzheimer disease,* and *Pick disease* are characterized by neuronal loss, cerebral cortical atrophy, and dementia. *Creutzfeldt-Jakob disease* is a dementia caused by prion disease and is morphologically characterized by spongiform degeneration of the brain. Higher mental functions are not seriously altered by multiple sclerosis.

29. **The answer is D.** Distal axonopathy is marked by *selective degeneration of the distal portion* of the axon and the surrounding myelin sheath. Schwann cells attempt to repair the damage and show reactive changes. Since the nucleus is not irreversibly damaged and the nerve cell is still viable, regeneration of the axon may take place through the formation of sprouts from the perikaryon.

30. **The answer is A.** Diabetes affects both the sensory and the motor portions of the peripheral nervous system and most often presents as *distal polyneuropathy.* Autonomic neuropathy and mononeuropathy are less common. The pathogenesis of these disorders is not fully understood, but they may be related to metabolic disturbances or to disease of small blood vessels. Vasculitis and paraproteinemia are not features of diabetes.

Chapter 29

The Eye

Questons

_____ 1. Inflammation of the eye, characterized by superficial hyperemia ("pink eye"), is in most instances best labeled as
   A. trachoma.
   B. keratitis.
   C. conjunctivitis.
   D. retinitis.
   E. glaucoma.

_____ 2. Seasonal recurrent conjunctivitis is most likely due to
   A. chemical irritation.
   B. autoimmune disease.
   C. exogenous allergens in the air.
   D. bacterial infection.
   E. viral infection.

_____ 3. Trachoma, the most common exogenous cause of blindness in parts of Africa and Middle East, is caused by
   A. virus.
   B. chlamydia.
   C. protozoa.
   D. fungi.
   E. autoimmune mechanisms.

_____ 4. All the following cause ophthalmia neonatorum _except_
   A. _Neisseria gonorrhoeae._
   B. _Chlamydia trachomatis._
   C. _Chlamydia oculogenitalis._
   D. _Staphylococcus aureus._
   E. _Onchocerca volvulus._

_____ 5. Melanoma of the eye usually originates from the
   A. cornea.
   B. sclera.
   C. lens.
   D. uvea.
   E. retina.

_____ **6.** In contrast to the skin, melanomas of the eye
  A. are not pigmented.
  B. are not malignant.
  C. do not metastasize primarily through the lymphatics.
  D. have a tendency to appear in childhood.
  E. rarely metastasize to the brain.

_____ **7.** Retinoblastomas are characterized by all the following *except*
  A. the peak incidence is in childhood.
  B. they may present with leukocoria (white pupil).
  C. they may be bilateral.
  D. they occur more commonly in some families.
  E. they are composed of giant cells.

_____ **8.** All the following apply to retinoblastomas *except*
  A. they tend to extend along the optic nerve.
  B. they invade blood vessels.
  C. they are fatal if untreated.
  D. only 30% of treated patients survive 5 years.
  E. they may be followed by other potentially fatal neoplasms, such as bone tumors.

_____ **9.** Siderosis bulbi is due to
  A. silica particles.
  B. a foreign body.
  C. microorganisms.
  D. predisposing metabolic disease.
  E. a bone fracture.

_____ **10.** All the following apply to "cotton-wool" patches in the retina *except*
  A. they are a consequence of hemorrhage.
  B. they are generally reversible.
  C. they consist of swollen axons in the nerve layer of retina.
  D. histologically, they contain cytoid bodies.
  E. the central retinal artery at the lamina cribrosa is often involved.

_____ **11.** Which of the following is true for central retinal vein occlusion?
  A. Less common than central artery occlusion
  B. Flame-shaped hemorrhages common
  C. Recovery poor
  D. Onset usually sudden
  E. Glaucoma uncommon

_____ **12.** "Cotton-wool spots," retinal hemorrhage, "macular star," edema of the optic nerve, and arterioverious nicking are indicative of
  A. central retinal vein occlusion.
  B. hypertension.
  C. pigmentary retinopathy.
  D. gangliosidosis.
  E. vitamin A deficiency.

_____ **13.** Diabetic retinopathy is
   A. more common in men than in women.
   B. more common in young diabetics than in old ones.
   C. a microangiopathy.
   D. inversely correlated with diabetic glomerulosclerosis.
   E. best treated with insulin.

_____ **14.** All the following are features of diabetic retinopathy *except*
   A. waxy exudates.
   B. capillary microaneurysms.
   C. neovascularization of the retina.
   D. retinal gliosis.
   E. retrolental fibroplasia.

_____ **15.** "Snowflake" cataracts in young diabetics develop because of
   A. lipid in the lens.
   B. lipid in the retina.
   C. glycogen in the iris.
   D. sorbitol in the lens.
   E. blood in the lens.

_____ **16.** Cataracts can be caused by
   A. metabolic disease.
   B. inflammation.
   C. drugs.
   D. all of the above.
   E. none of the above.

_____ **17.** The most common form of glaucoma in the United States is
   A. congenital.
   B. primary open angle.
   C. primary closed angle.
   D. low tension.
   E. secondary.

_____ **18.** The effects of glaucoma in adults include all the following *except*
   A. cupping of the optic disc.
   B. optic atrophy.
   C. degeneration of the ganglion cell layer in the retina.
   D. bulging sclera and cornea.
   E. buphthalmos.

_____ **19.** Retinal detachment may be caused by
   A. retinal degeneration.
   B. intraocular hemorrhage.
   C. vitreoretinal adhesions.
   D. none of the above.
   E. all of the above.

_____ **20.** Retinitis pigmentosa, or progressive degenerative retinopathy, may be
   A. autosomal dominant retinal disease.
   B. autosomal recessive retinal disease.
   C. X-linked recessive disease.
   D. part of a systemic disease.
   E. all of the above.

_____ **21.** Edema of the optic disc ("papilledema") is a reliable sign of
   A. cerebral edema.
   B. dehydration.
   C. carotenemia.
   D. liver disease.
   E. kidney disease.

_____ **22.** Myopia is usually associated with
   A. increased anteroposterior diameter of the eye.
   B. glaucoma.
   C. retinal degeneration.
   D. cataract.
   E. optic nerve atrophy.

Answers

1. **The answer is C.** Hyperemia of the external ocular blood vessels is mostly due to conjunctival inflammation (conjunctivitis). The inflammatory exudate may accumulate in the conjunctival sac, causing pain, swelling, and inability to open the eyes.

2. **The answer is C.** Seasonal conjunctivitis is typically caused by allergies to pollen.

3. **The answer is B.** Trachoma is caused by *Chlamydia trachomatis,* an infectious agent that causes bilateral eye infection in underdeveloped countries with poor hygiene. In children the disease usually heals spontaneously. In adults it may cause blindness, especially if combined with superinfection.

4. **The answer is E.** *Onchocerca volvulus,* an important cause of blindness in Africa and Latin America, is a nematode transmitted by black flies. It is not acquired at birth and is not susceptible to antibiotic eye drops. All other organisms listed may be transmitted to the newborn from the mother at the time of delivery, and infection is prevented by antibiotic eye drops.

5. **The answer is D.** Melanocytes are found in both the uvea and the retina, but the retinal melanocytes do not undergo malignant transformation as readily as those in the uvea. The *choroid* is the most common site of origin of ocular melanomas.

6. **The answer is C.** Uvea melanomas are composed of melanocytes. Similar to the situation in the skin, they may be heavily pigmented or amelanotic. Melanomas are malignant irrespective of their site of origin. Ocular melanomas *do not metastasize through lymphatics*, because the eye does not have lymphatics. Again, similar to melanomas of the skin, they do not appear in children. Metastases to the brain are not uncommon in disseminated tumors.

7. **The answer is E.** Retinoblastoma typically occurs in children. In 25% of sporadic cases and in most of the familial cases, the tumors are bilateral. Because the tumor is pale it produces a white pupil and the so-called cat's eye reflex. Histologically, these tumors are composed of small retinal cell precursors. Retinoblastoma is one of the typical "small blue cell

tumors" of infancy and childhood, similar to neuroblastoma or medulloblastoma, to which it is related. *Giant cells are not a feature of retinoblastoma.*

8. **The answer is D.** Retinoblastoma has a *favorable prognosis*. If detected early and treated properly, 90% of children survive more than 5 years. However, it is generally fatal if untreated. Metastases occur either along the optic nerve or through the blood vessels. Patients treated for retinoblastoma often develop other tumors during adolescence, such as osteogenic sarcoma, Ewing sarcoma, or pineoblastoma.

9. **The answer is B.** Siderosis bulbi may occur several years after an iron-containing *foreign body* has lodged in the eye. Oxidation of the iron causes a rusty discoloration of the ocular tissues.

10. **The answer is A.** "Cotton-wool" patches are typically a consequence of arterial occlusive disease in the retina and *are not due to hemorrhage*. The changes in the axons, which histologically appear as cytoid bodies, are reversible. Emboli most often lodge in the central retinal artery in the lamina cribrosa (i.e., the point where the sclera is perforate for the passage of the optic nerve).

11. **The answer is B.** Central retinal vein occlusion is more common than occlusion of the retinal artery. It typically evolves gradually and has a better prognosis. Funduscopic examination usually reveals *flame-shaped hemorrhages*. The intraocular pressure tends to be elevated.

12. **The answer is B.** A combination of ischemic changes and hemorrhages in the retina, combined with arteriovenous nicking, is typical of *hypertension*. Pigmentary retinopathy occurs because of several inborn errors of metabolism, vitamin A deficiency, certain drugs, and inflammation.

13. **The answer is C.** Diabetic retinopathy is a consequence of *microvascular disease* and correlates with glomerular disease. Similar to diabetes in general, it is more common in women. Retinopathy is a consequence of longstanding diabetes and usually develops 20 to 30 years after the onset of the disease. Once ocular vasculopathy has developed, it can be treated by focal photocoagulation. Although good control of diabetes may retard the development of diabetic retinopathy, insulin treatment has no effect on established vascular lesions.

14. **The answer is E.** *Retrolental fibroplasia* is an iatrogenic disease in premature infants caused by exposure to high concentrations of oxygen. Waxy exudates, capillary microaneurysms, and gliosis, with consequent detachment of the retina, characterize proliferative retinopathy.

15. **The answer is D.** In diabetes, a cataract develops in the lens because of the accumulation of *sorbitol*, an alcohol derived from the metabolism of glucose. The accumulation of glycogen in the iris causes lacy vacuolization, and lipemia retinalis accounts for the waxy streaks seen by funduscopy. Bleeding occurs in the cornea and vitreous body and can cause glaucoma, owing to the formation of anterior synechiae.

16. **The answer is D.** A "cataract" (i.e., an opacity of the lens) may have *numerous causes*. It can be caused by ocular as well as systemic diseases. The cause may not always be obvious, as in older persons (senile cataract).

17. **The answer is B.** *Primary open-angle glaucoma* is a disease of old age that affects 1% to 3% of the population over 40 years of age. It is almost always bilateral and develops insidiously. The elevation of intraocular pressure may initially cause the loss of peripheral vision. If untreated, glaucoma eventually leads to blindness. The angle of the anterior chamber is apparently normal, but there is increased resistance to the flow of aqueous humor in the vicinity of Schlemm's canal. Myopia and diabetes increase the risk of this form of glaucoma.

18. **The answer is E.** *Buphthalmos* ("ox eye") occurs only in children, because in adults the rigid sclera prevents generalized enlargement of the eye. The increased intraocular pressure causes bulging at weak points and cupping of the optic disc. Compression atrophy of the optic nerve and ganglion cells accounts for the problems with vision.

19. **The answer is E.** Retinal detachment can be caused by a *number of retinal and other eye disorders* that cause separation of the sensory retina from the retinal pigmentary epithelium.

20. **The answer is E.** Retinitis pigmentosa is a generic term that denotes a group of retinal diseases that share the same morphologic manifestations. These conditions include several *inherited* retionopathies and metabolic disorders (e.g., cystinosis or mucopolysaccharidoses). Retinitis pigmentosa may also be a consequence of various *inflammatory conditions*, such as syphilis or rubella infection.

21. **The answer is A.** Papilledema is a reliable sign of *cerebral edema*. Although it may also occur in hepatic and renal disease, owing to generalized edema and fluid retention, this situation is not common.

22. **The answer is A.** More than 70 million people in this country are nearsighted (myopic). In myopia, light entering the eye is focused anterior to the retina, owing to a longer than usual *anteroposterior diameter* of the eye.

Final Examination

_____ 1. Agenesis of ganglion cells should be confirmed histologically for the diagnosis of
A. congenital pyloric stenosis.
B. Hirschsprung disease.
C. vesicoureteric reflux.
D. achalasia of the esophagus.
E. toxic megacolon.

_____ 2. Which of the following is a constant feature of all forms of cirrhosis?
A. Fat in hepatocytes
B. Fibrous scars
C. Deposits of iron
D. Mallory's hyaline
E. Enlargement of the liver

_____ 3. A lung tumor composed of neuroendocrine cells is called
A. small cell (oat cell) carcinoma.
B. adenocarcinoma.
C. squamous cell carcinoma.
D. mesothelioma.
E. bronchioloalveolar carcinoma.

_____ 4. Anemia of thalassemia minor is a consequence of
A. intrinsic factor deficiency.
B. iron deficiency.
C. metabolic inhibition of DNA replication.
D. a gene defect.
E. hemolytic crisis.

_____ 5. Elevated levels of 5-hydroxyindolacetic and (5-HIAA) are most helpful in the diagnosis of
A. polyposis coli.
B. endometriosis.
C. lymphoma.
D. neuroblastoma.
E. hepatocellular carcinoma.

_____ 6. Microcytic hypochromic anemia is a common complication of
A. menopause.
B. menorrhagia.
C. amenorrhea.
D. endometriosis.
E. chronic vaginitis.

_____ 7. The adrenogenital syndrome in infants is caused by
A. pituitary tumor.
B. congenital adrenal tumor.
C. inborn error of metabolism.
D. Leydig cell tumor.
E. deficiency of hepatic conjugation of androstenedione.

_____ 8. Macrocytic anemia that responds to administration of intrinsic factor is associated with
A. chronic liver disease.
B. blind intestinal loop syndrome.
C. duodenal ulcer.
D. atrophic gastritis.
E. hypertrophic gastritis.

_____ 9. In which of the following conditions is steatorrhea not a characteristic finding?
A. Cystic fibrosis
B. Whipple disease
C. Peptic ulcer disease
D. Chronic pancreatitis
E. Celiac disease

_____ 10. Most testicular tumors originate from
A. germ cells.
B. Sertoli cells.
C. spermatozoa.
D. Leydig cells.
E. sex cord sustentacular cells.

_____ 11. Primary mucus-secreting carcinomas occur most often in the
A. esophagus.
B. lung.
C. liver.
D. colon.
E. small intestine.

_____ 12. What is the most common site of origin of neuroblastoma in young children and infants?
A. Brain
B. Cerebellum
C. Peripheral nerves
D. Mediastinal paraganglia
E. Adrenal

_____ 13. Squamous cell carcinoma of the lung presents most commonly with symptoms related to
A. bronchial irritation.
B. inappropriate hormone production.
C. bone metastases.
D. compression of the superior vena cava.
E. obstruction of the pulmonary artery.

_____ **14.** Which of the following diseases causes group atrophy of muscle fibers?
  A. Amyotrophic lateral sclerosis
  B. Multiple sclerosis
  C. Subacute combined degeneration
  D. Duchenne muscular dystrophy
  E. Myositis

_____ **15.** Signet ring carcinoma metastatic to supraclavicular lymph nodes originates most often from the
  A. thyroid.
  B. lung.
  C. stomach.
  D. small intestine.
  E. esophagus.

_____ **16.** Cretinism is a consequence of neonatal deficiency of
  A. magnesium.
  B. iodine.
  C. calcium.
  D. fluoride.
  E. vitamin E.

_____ **17.** Most primary intracranial tumors originate from
  A. neurons.
  B. astrocytes.
  C. oligodendroglia.
  D. microglia.
  E. ependymal lining cells.

_____ **18.** The least common secondary change in a leiomyoma of the uterus is
  A. malignant transformation.
  B. calcification.
  C. infarction.
  D. hyalinization.
  E. torsion with hemorrhagic necrosis.

_____ **19.** Which of the following tumors has the best prognosis?
  A. Squamous cell carcinoma of the bronchus
  B. Adenocarcinoma of the lung
  C. Small cell undifferentiated carcinoma of the lung
  D. Squamous cell carcinoma of the larynx
  E. Mesothelioma

_____ **20.** Multiple radiolucent "punched-out" lesions of bone associated with Bence-Jones protein in the urine are most often associated with
  A. hyperamylasemia.
  B. hypercalcemia.
  C. hyperkalemia.
  D. hyponatremia.
  E. hyperglycemia.

_____ **21.** All the following statements are true about carcinoma of the head of the pancreas *except*
  A. it is the most common location of carcinoma of the pancreas.
  B. jaundice is a common presenting symptom.
  C. it metastasizes to regional lymph nodes.
  D. it is usually inoperable.
  E. it is hormonally active.

_____ **22.** Lack of surfactant in the pulmonary alveoli causes
  A. pneumonia.
  B. emphysema.
  C. atelectasis.
  D. pleuritis.
  E. interstitial fibrosis.

_____ **23.** Fibroadenomas of the breasts are typically
  A. premalignant lesions.
  B. composed of fibrous tissue and highly atypical epithelium.
  C. found in postmenopausal women.
  D. composed of sarcomatous stroma and regular cuboidal epithelium.
  E. well circumscribed.

_____ **24.** All of the following lesions produce pulmonary metastases *except*
  A. choriocarcinoma.
  B. hydatidiform mole.
  C. leiomyosarcoma of uterus.
  D. embryonal carcinoma of the ovary.
  E. ovarian serous cystadenocarcinoma.

_____ **25.** Arthritis is a recognized extraintestinal manifestation of
  A. abetalipoproteinemia.
  B. celiac disease.
  C. Crohn disease.
  D. Meckel diverticulum.
  E. diverticulosis of the colon.

_____ **26.** Tetralogy of Fallot includes all the following *except*
  A. dextroposition of aorta.
  B. pulmonary artery stenosis.
  C. ventricular septal defect.
  D. hypertrophy of the right ventricle.
  E. atrial septal defect.

_____ **27.** Which is the most common cause of death in leukemia?
  A. Aplastic anemia
  B. Disseminated infection
  C. Hemorrhage into the brain
  D. Hyperviscosity of the blood
  E. Rupture of the spleen

_____ **28.** Retinoblastomas develop due to gene
   A. deletion.
   B. amplification.
   C. aberrant activation.
   D. translocation.
   E. transposition.

_____ **29.** Uniform granular ("lumpy-bumpy") deposits of immunoglobu-
   lin in glomeruli are diagnostic of
   A. nephrotic syndrome.
   B. glomerulonephritis mediated by immune complexes.
   C. glomerulonephritis induced by antibody to glomerular base-
   ment membrane.
   D. pyelonephritis.
   E. glomerular lesion induced by malignant hypertension.

_____ **30.** Which of the following is the least common complication of
   myocardial infarction?
   A. Cardiac arrhythmia
   B. Mural thrombus
   C. Cardiac rupture
   D. Cardiac failure
   E. Fibrinous pericarditis

_____ **31.** Which of the following diseases is not considered to predispose
   to atherosclerosis?
   A. Diabetes
   B. Familial hyperlipidemia
   C. Hypothyroidism
   D. Chronic nephrotic syndrome
   E. Cirrhosis

_____ **32.** All of the following are associated with cirrhosis *except*
   A. increased incidence of hepatocellular carcinoma.
   B. hepatorenal syndrome.
   C. gastrointestinal hemorrhage.
   D. jaundice.
   E. migratory thrombophlebitis.

_____ **33.** Malabsorption is a complication of all the following *except*
   A. chronic pancreatitis.
   B. carcinoma of the rectum.
   C. biliary tract obstruction.
   D. scleroderma.
   E. abetalipoproteinemia.

_____ **34.** Consequences and complications of arterial hypertension
   include all of the following *except*
   A. left ventricular hypertrophy.
   B. accelerated atherosclerosis.
   C. intracerebral hemorrhage.
   D. ocular papilledema.
   E. paradoxical embolism.

_____ **35.** Myotonic dystrophy is
A. inherited as a sex-linked recessive trait.
B. associated with neonatal symptoms.
C. marked by elevated serum creatine kinase.
D. more common in women than men.
E. invariably lethal in adolescence.

_____ **36.** Membranoproliferative glomerulonephritis type I is character-
ized by all of the following *except*
A. low serum complement.
B. hematuria.
C. proteinuria.
D. peripheral edema.
E. epithelial crescents in two-thirds of the glomeruli.

_____ **37.** All of the following are true of primary biliary cirrhosis *except*
A. it affects women more than men.
B. it causes hepatic fibrosis.
C. it causes stenosis of the common bile duct.
D. it presents with antimitochondrial antibodies in the serum.
E. it is associated with autoimmune diseases.

_____ **38.** Besides the skin melanoma most often develops in the
A. substantia nigra of the brain.
B. choroid plexus.
C. eye.
D. ear.
E. olfactory nerve.

_____ **39.** Decreased synthesis of lipoproteins in alcoholic liver injury is a
cause of
A. formation of alcoholic hyaline.
B. fatty change of hepatocytes.
C. hemosiderosis.
D. hepatic fibrosis.
E. increased gluconeogenesis.

_____ **40.** Which of the following will most likely involve the rectum?
A. Ulcerative colitis
B. Cholera
C. Tuberculous colitis
D. Ischemic colitis
E. Salmonellosis

_____ **41.** The pathologic changes of acute pancreatitis include all of the
following *except*
A. edema.
B. fat necrosis.
C. hemorrhage.
D. necrosis of pancreatic acini.
E. intraductal mucous plugs in the small pancreatic ducts.

_____ **42.** Tumors causing the syndrome of watery diarrhea, hypokalemia, and achlorhydria are most often located in the
A. stomach.
B. pancreas.
C. liver.
D. ileum.
E. colon.

_____ **43.** All of the following are common in systemic lupus erythematosus *except*
A. skin rash.
B. myocarditis.
C. joint disease.
D. anemia.
E. glomerulonephritis.

_____ **44.** Which of the following tumors most often secretes a parathyroid hormone related peptide (PTHrP) causing hypercalcemia?
A. Squamous cell carcinoma of bronchus
B. Medullary carcinoma of thyroid
C. Medullary carcinoma of the breast
D. Medulloblastoma
E. Granulosa cell tumor of the ovary

_____ **45.** Neuroendocrine granules are seen in all the following tumors *except*
A. pheochromocytoma.
B. neuroblastoma.
C. islet cell carcinoma.
D. carcinoid.
E. Leydig cell tumor.

_____ **46.** All of the following lesions are associated with asbestosis *except*
A. carcinoma of the lung.
B. mesothelioma.
C. asthma.
D. interstitial pulmonary fibrosis.
E. pleural fibrous plaques.

_____ **47.** Esophagitis is associated with all the following *except*
A. ectopic gastric mucosa.
B. hiatal hernia.
C. reflux of gastric juices into the esophagus.
D. scleroderma.
E. pernicious anemia.

_____ **48.** Hypertension in a 35-year-old man with bilaterally enlarged kidneys is most likely caused by
A. Wilms tumor.
B. polycystic renal disease.
C. amyloidosis.
D. chronic glomerulonephritis.
E. chronic pyelonephritis.

_____ **49.** Membranous nephropathy may be associated with all the following *except*
A. diabetes.
B. systemic lupus erythematosus.
C. malignant tumor.
D. hepatitis B.
E. syphilis.

_____ **50.** Which of the following hormones may cause peptic ulcer?
A. Corticosteroids
B. Thyroid hormones
C. Follicle stimulating hormone (FSH)
D. Prolactin
E. Estrogen

_____ **51.** Acute poststreptococcal glomerulonephritis is associated with all the following *except*
A. hematuria.
B. hypertension.
C. red cell casts.
D. decreased serum complement.
E. hyperlipidemia.

_____ **52.** Berylliosis is characterized by
A. granulomas.
B. pigmentation of the lung parenchyma.
C. particles visible only by polarized microscopy.
D. exposure to quartz.
E. mesothelioma as a common complication.

_____ **53.** Saccular aneurysms due to congenital weakness of the vessel wall are most often found in the
A. abdominal aorta.
B. ascending aorta.
C. thoracic aorta.
D. circle of Willis.
E. arteries of the upper extremities.

_____ **54.** Which of the following has the same histologic features as mucinous cystadenocarcinoma of the ovary?
A. Carcinoma of the cervix
B. Carcinoma of the endometrium
C. Carcinoid
D. Renal cell carcinoma
E. Colon cancer

_____ **55.** An expanded sella turcica seen by x-ray may be a feature of
A. acromegaly.
B. hyperaldosteronism.
C. adrenogenital syndrome.
D. Zollinger-Ellison syndrome.
E. osteitis fibrosa cystica.

_____ **56.** Gumma is a feature of
  A. silicosis.
  B. sarcoidosis.
  C. tuberculosis.
  D. syphilis.
  E. histoplasmosis.

_____ **57.** Splenomegaly is common in terminal stages of all the following diseases *except*
  A. chronic lymphocytic leukemia.
  B. chronic myelogenous leukemia.
  C. spherocytosis.
  D. sickle cell anemia.
  E. Hodgkin's disease, stage IV.

_____ **58.** All of the following statements about ventricular septal defects are true *except*
  A. intramembranous defect is more common than intramuscular defect.
  B. it is often associated with other heart defects.
  C. it is relatively common in comparison with other congenital heart disorders.
  D. it is a possible route for paradoxical emboli.
  E. initially, the shunting of blood through the defect is almost always right to left.

_____ **59.** All of the following statements regarding carcinoma of the cervix are true *except* that
  A. it is associated with human papillomavirus infection.
  B. squamous cell carcinoma is the most common type.
  C. the peak incidence occurs between the ages of 20 and 30.
  D. it can be detected by vaginal exfoliative cytology.
  E. if untreated it can be fatal.

_____ **60.** Infertility is a complication of all the following *except*
  A. polycystic ovary syndrome.
  B. cryptorchidism.
  C. klinefelter syndrome.
  D. Turner syndrome.
  E. trichomonas vaginalis infection.

_____ **61.** Which of the following lesions shows the most prominent cyclic hormonal changes during the normal menstrual cycle?
  A. Carcinoma of the cervix
  B. Endometriosis of the fallopian tube
  C. Thecoma of the ovary
  D. Pseudomyxoma peritonei
  E. Condyloma acuminatum

_____ **62.** Cor pulmonale is a well-recognized complication of all of the following *except*
  A. silicosis.
  B. pulmonary emphysema.
  C. mitral stenosis.
  D. mitral insufficiency.
  E. endocarditis of the tricuspid valve.

_____ **63.** Vaginal bleeding is a common symptom of all the following
except
   A. endometrial hyperplasia.
   B. adenocarcinoma of the endometrium.
   C. carcinoma in situ of the uterine cervix.
   D. endometrial polyp.
   E. hydrosalpinx.

_____ **64.** All of the following are characteristic of prostatic carcinoma
except
   A. it is more common in older men.
   B. it metastasizes to bone.
   C. it is an adenocarcinoma.
   D. it secretes tumor markers in serum.
   E. it responds favorably to hormonal therapy.

_____ **65.** All of the following organs are more likely to be affected by
metastatic tumors than by primary tumors *except*
   A. liver.
   B. lung.
   C. uterus.
   D. adrenals.
   E. mediastinal lymph nodes.

_____ **66.** Hyperplasia of bronchial glands occurs in all the following
except
   A. chronic bronchitis.
   B. cystic fibrosis.
   C. extrinsic asthma.
   D. intrinsic asthma.
   E. α-1 antitrypsin deficiency.

_____ **67.** Polyps occur in all of the following *except*
   A. colon.
   B. urinary bladder.
   C. endometrium.
   D. liver.
   E. stomach.

_____ **68.** Which of the following infectious agents will produce changes in
the epithelial cell nuclei of the cervix recognizable in a pap
smear?
   A. Herpesvirus
   B. Syphilis
   C. Gonorrhea
   D. Human immunodeficiency virus
   E. Trichomonas vaginalis

_____ **69.** Fibrotic nodules rich in birefringent crystals are typically found
in lungs affected by
   A. anthracosis.
   B. silicosis.
   C. asbestosis.
   D. sarcoidosis.
   E. tuberculosis.

_____ **70.** There is an increased incidence of duodenal peptic ulcer in patients with all the following *except*
A. cirrhosis.
B. Zollinger-Ellison syndrome.
C. renal transplants.
D. multiple endocrine neoplasia syndrome type 1.
E. pernicious anemia.

_____ **71.** Neonatal meningitis is most often caused by
A. *Hemophilus influenzae.*
B. *Streptococcus pneumoniae.*
C. *Neisseria meningitidis.*
D. *Escherichia coli.*
E. *Staphylococcus aureus.*

_____ **72.** Hemorrhage in the internal capsule of the brain is most often associated with
A. endocarditis.
B. berry aneurysm.
C. hypertension.
D. sepsis.
E. cardiogenic shock.

_____ **73.** All of the following features characterize glioblastoma multiforme *except*
A. infiltrative growth.
B. widespread areas of necrosis.
C. characteristic vascular changes.
D. poor prognosis.
E. invasion of cranial bones.

_____ **74.** Hyperviscosity of the blood is a feature of
A. hypercalcemia.
B. hyperlipidemia.
C. hyperglobulinemia.
D. hyperammonemia.
E. hyperuricemia.

_____ **75.** Osteopenia may be caused by all of the following *except*
A. primary hyperparathyroidism.
B. secondary hyperparathyroidism.
C. end-stage Paget disease of bone.
D. adrenal corticosteroids.
E. osteoporosis.

_____ **76.** Huntington disease is associated with
A. chromosomal changes.
B. autosomal dominant inheritance.
C. microscopic signs of chronic inflammation.
D. senile plaques.
E. slow virus infection.

_____ 77. Which of the following is the most typical reaction to infection with *Mycobacterium tuberculosis*?
A. Hemorrhage
B. Fibrinoid degeneration
C. Caseous necrosis
D. Pus formation
E. Abscess formation

_____ 78. Volvulus most often involves the
A. cecum.
B. ascending colon.
C. transverse colon.
D. sigmoid colon.
E. rectum.

_____ 79. Which of the following is a prominent feature of hay fever?
A. Increase in nasal tissue
B. Lymphocytosis
C. Lack of reactivity to allergens injected into the skin
D. Anemia
E. Monoclonal immunoglobulin peak in serum electrophoresis

_____ 80. All of the following diseases are more common in women than in men *except*
A. Graves disease.
B. rheumatoid arthritis.
C. primary biliary cirrhosis.
D. goodpasture syndrome.
E. cholecystitis.

_____ 81. Which of the following diseases is caused by genetic defects involving the gene for Duchenne muscular dystrophy?
A. Becker muscular dystrophy
B. Scapulohumeral muscular dystrophy
C. Myotonic muscular dystrophy
D. Myasthenia gravis
E. Werdnig-Hoffman disease

_____ 82. Patchy necrosis of the colonic mucosa covered with crusts of fibrin and cell detritus is caused by
A. *Campylobacter jejuni.*
B. *E. coli.*
C. *Clostridium difficile.*
D. Shigella.
E. Herpes simplex virus, type 1.

_____ 83. Benign tumors in the cerebellopontine angle usually originate from
A. facial nerve.
B. olfactory nerve.
C. acoustic nerve.
D. cerebellum.
E. pons.

_____ 84. All of the following are typical features of multiple sclerosis *except*
A. demyelination of white matter.
B. lesions of the optic nerve.
C. lesions in the white matter of the spinal cord.
D. oligoclonal immunoglobulin bands in cerebrospinal fluid.
E. laminar necrosis of the cerebral cortex.

_____ 85. Viral encephalitis is characterized by
A. Alzheimer type II astrocytes.
B. lymphocytic infiltrates in perivascular Virchow-Robin spaces.
C. aggregates of neutrophils in the cerebral cortex.
D. plasma cells diffusely infiltrating the white substance of the brain.
E. microabscesses.

_____ 86. Which of the following lesions is a complication of diabetes mellitus?
A. Berry aneurysm of the circle of Willis
B. Centrolobular sclerosis of the liver
C. Intralobular sclerosis of the breast
D. Papillary necrosis of the kidney
E. Budd-Chiari syndrome

_____ 87. Chronic myelogenous leukemia is usually associated with all of the following *except*
A. infections.
B. migratory thrombophlebitis.
C. decreased neutrophilic alkaline phosphatase.
D. splenomegaly.
E. anemia.

_____ 88. Typical features of fibrocystic change of the breast include all the following *except*
A. cystic dilation of ducts.
B. intraductal papillomas.
C. interstitial fibrosis.
D. ductal hyperplasia.
E. galactorrhea-amenorrhea.

_____ 89. Most testicular tumors
A. are malignant.
B. occur predominantly in elderly men.
C. secrete androgens.
D. present with symptoms related to distant metastases.
E. produce hematogenous metastases more often than lymphatic metastases.

_____ 90. Both Cushing syndrome and pheochromocytoma may be associated with
A. hypertension.
B. osteoporosis.
C. alkalosis.
D. abdominal striae
E. excessive accumulation of subcutaneous fat.

_____ 91. Which is the most common tumor of long bones of the extremities in the elderly?
   A. Liposarcoma
   B. Ewing sarcoma
   C. Metastatic carcinoma
   D. Osteogenic sarcoma
   E. Chondrosarcoma

_____ 92. The most common cause of hyperthyroidism is
   A. enzyme deficiency.
   B. autoimmunity.
   C. bacterial infection.
   D. viral infection.
   E. tumor.

_____ 93. A cystic cavity in the pancreas filled with turbid brownish yellow fluid is most likely a
   A. mucinous cystadenoma.
   B. follicular cyst.
   C. pseudocyst.
   D. cystic fibrosis.
   E. dermoid cyst.

_____ 94. All of the following statements about Reed-Sternberg cells are true *except*
   A. they are larger than plasma cells.
   B. they have prominent nucleoli.
   C. they have a bilobed nucleus.
   D. they are rich in terminal deoxynucleotidyl transferase.
   E. they occur in lymph nodes and extranodal lesions.

_____ 95. All of the following predispose to the formation of varicose veins of the lower extremities *except*
   A. pregnancy.
   B. heart failure.
   C. congenital weakness of connective tissue.
   D. Raynaud disease.
   E. thrombophlebitis.

_____ 96. Typical features of mitral stenosis include all the following *except*
   A. left atrial dilation.
   B. left ventricular hypertrophy.
   C. pulmonary alveolar hemorrhages.
   D. pulmonary hypertension.
   E. mitral calcification.

_____ 97. The major manifestations of rheumatic fever include all the following *except*
   A. chorea.
   B. pancarditis.
   C. subcutaneous nodules.
   D. ankylosing spondylitis.
   E. arthritis.

_____ **98.** Stenosis or partial occlusion of one renal artery would most likely cause
A. hypertension.
B. pyuria.
C. hematuria.
D. proteinuria.
E. oliguria.

_____ **99.** Loss of renal parenchyma in the elderly is most often a consequence of
A. acute glomerulonephritis.
B. nephrosclerosis due to atherosclerosis.
C. chronic pyelonephritis.
D. renal vein thrombosis.
E. nephrolithiasis.

_____ **100.** All of the following intracranial neoplasms could present as an infratentorial mass *except*
A. cerebellar astrocytoma.
B. schwannoma.
C. craniopharyngioma.
D. meningioma.
E. medulloblastoma.

_____ **101.** Primary tumors of the spinal cord include all the following *except*
A. astrocytoma.
B. glioblastoma multiforme.
C. medulloblastoma.
D. ependymoma.
E. lymphoma.

A n s w e r s

1. **The answer is C.** *Vesicoureteric reflux.* Hirschsprung disease is a congenital disorder characterized by an absence of ganglion cells in the rectum. The diagnosis is established by biopsy, which shows that the constricted portion of the large intestine does not contain ganglion cells. See Chapter 13.

2. **The answer is B.** *Fibrous scars.* Fibrosis is a constant feature in all forms of cirrhosis. See Chapter 14.

3. **The answer is A.** *Small cell (oat cell) carcinoma.* Small cell (oat cell) carcinoma of the lung is composed of neuroendocrine cells. These tumor cells contain typical neuroendocrine granules visible by electron microscopy and react with antibodies to polypeptide hormones normally found in bronchial neuroendocrine cells. See Chapter 12.

4. **The answer is D.** *A gene defect.* Thalassemia syndromes are a heterogeneous group of heritable anemias related to a mutation in the alpha or beta globin gene. See Chapter 20.

5. **The answer is D.** *Neuroblastoma.* Elevated levels of 5-hydroxyindolacetic acid (5-HIAA) are typically found in patients with neuroblastoma. 5-HIAA vanillylmandelic acid (VMA) and homovanillic acid are cate-cholamines derived from other catecholamines, epinephrine, and norep-inephrine secreted by the tumor cells. Pheochromocytoma, which also originates from the adrenal medulla, is also characterized by elevated levels of catecholamines in serum and urine. See Chapter 21.

6. **The answer is B.** *Menorrhagia.* Menorrhagia (i.e., severe menstrual bleed-ing) results in excessive blood loss and depletion of body iron stores. If the iron stores are not restored, iron deficiency anemia ensues. Iron defi-ciency anemia is microcytic and hypochromic. See Chapter 20.

7. **The answer is C.** *Inborn error of metabolism.* The adrenogenital syndrome in infants is caused by an inborn error of metabolism, which results in adrenal cortical hyperplasia and hypersecretion of androgens. A muta-tion in the gene encoding the enzyme 21-hydroxylase accounts for more than 90% of all the cases. See Chapters 17 and 21.

8. **The answer is D.** *Atrophic gastritis.* Macrocytic anemia that responds to intrinsic factor therapy is a form of pernicious anemia that is typically associated with atrophic gastritis. In such patients vitamin B_{12} cannot be absorbed from the intestinal tract because the atrophic gastric mucosa does not secrete intrinsic factor, which binds to vitamin B_{12} and is essen-tial for its absorption in the ileum. See Chapters 13 and 20.

9. **The answer is C.** *Peptic ulcer disease.* Steatorrhea (i.e., fatty bulky stools) is not a feature of peptic ulcer disease, because peptic ulcer does not adversely affect fat absorption in the small intestine. See Chapter 13.

10. **The answer is A.** *Germ cells.* Most testicular tumors (95%) originate from germ cells. The remaining 5% arise from the sex cord cells, Sertoli and Leydig cells, or nonspecific connective-tissue stromal cells (e.g., fibro-blasts, smooth muscle cells). Rare tumors represent metastases from some other primary site. See Chapter 17.

11. **The answer is D.** *Colon.* The colon is the most common site of origin of mucus-secreting adenocarcinomas. Small intestinal cancers are uncom-mon. See Chapter 13.

12. **The answer is E.** *Adrenal.* Neuroblastomas can originate from any site that contains derivatives of migratory neural crest cells. The adrenal medulla is the most common site of origin of neuroblastomas in young children and infants. Neuroblastomas may also originate from extra-adrenal paraganglia of the abdominal and thoracic cavity, which are typ-ically located around the aorta. The central nervous system is a rare source of neuroblastomas. See Chapter 21.

13. **The answer is A.** *Bronchial irritation.* Squamous cell carcinoma of the lung originates most often from the major bronchi and presents with coughing and expectoration indicative of bronchial irritation. See Chap-ter 12.

14. **The answer is A.** *Amyotrophic lateral sclerosis.* Amyotrophic lateral scle-rosis is a disease of the upper (cortical) or lower (spinal) motor neurons. Loss of these motor neurons results in denervation atrophy of skeletal muscles, which typically affects groups of muscle fibers. See Chapters 27 and 28.

15. **The answer is C.** *Stomach.* Signet ring carcinoma in a supraclavicular lymph node (known as Virchow's node) is most often a metastasis from a primary gastric adenocarcinoma. Less commonly, mucinous carcinomas from the intestines, gall bladder, or pancreas may also reach the supraclavicular lymph nodes through the lymphatic routes (thoracic duct). See Chapter 13.

16. **The answer is B.** *Iodine.* Lack of iodine results in thyroid insufficiency, which may adversely affect the normal development of the brain and somatic growth. Cretinism is characterized by mental retardation and short stature. See Chapter 21.

17. **The answer is B.** *Astrocytes.* Glioblastoma multiforme and astrocytoma, the most common primary brain tumors, originate from astrocytes. See Chapter 28.

18. **The answer is A.** *Malignant transformation.* Leiomyomas of the uterus rarely undergo malignant transformation. Uterine leiomyosarcomas typically originate de novo and not from preexisting benign tumors. See Chapter 18.

19. **The answer is D.** *Squamous cell carcinoma of the larynx.* Squamous cell carcinoma of the larynx has a relatively good prognosis. Glottic tumors are slowly growing lesions, most of which can be cured by surgery or radiation therapy. Supraglottic and infraglottic tumors are more aggressive, and at least 30% of patients have local metastases at the time of operation. Even so, laryngeal carcinoma has a better prognosis than the other cancers listed. See Chapter 25.

20. **The answer is B.** *Hypercalcemia.* Multiple radiolucent punched-out bone lesions associated with Bence-Jones protein are features of multiple myeloma, which is typically associated with hypercalcemia. Hypercalcemia results from the release of calcium from the destroyed bone. See Chapters 20 and 26.

21. **The answer is E.** *It is hormonally active.* Carcinoma of the pancreas is not hormonally active because these tumors originate from the exocrine rather than the endocrine cells of the pancreas. See Chapter 15.

22. **The answer is C.** *Atelectasis.* Lack of surfactant in the lungs of premature infants causes atelectasis. See Chapter 6.

23. **The answer is E.** *Well-circumscribed.* Fibroadenomas of the breast are well-circumscribed benign tumors, typically found in young women. They are not premalignant and contain no sarcomatous elements. See Chapter 19.

24. **The answer is B.** *Hydatidiform mole.* Hydatidiform mole is a placental lesion related to chromosomal abnormalities in the conceptus. It is not a neoplasm, and it does not metastasize. All the other tumors listed can metastasize to the lungs. See Chapter 18.

25. **The answer is C.** *Crohn disease.* Arthritis is an uncommon but well-known extraintestinal complication of Crohn disease. See Chapter 13.

26. **The answer is E.** *Atrial septal defect.* All the other abnormalities listed are typical features of tetralogy of Fallot, which does not affect the atrium and does not cause atrial septal defects. See Chapter 11.

27. **The answer is B.** *Disseminated infection.* Patients suffering from leukemia die most often of overwhelming infections. Leukemic patients lose the capacity to produce normal leukocytes, which are essential for combatting bacterial and fungal infections. Cytotoxic therapy used in the treatment of leukemia further diminishes normal hemopoiesis. See Chapter 20.

28. **The answer is A.** *Deletion.* Retinoblastoma is a tumor of infancy and childhood that develops because of the deletion of a segment of the long arm of chromosome 13 that contains the Rb tumor suppressor gene. See Chapters 5, 6, and 29.

29. **The answer is B.** *Glomerulonephritis mediated by immune complexes.* Uniform, granular ("lumpy-bumpy") deposits of immunoglobulin along the glomerular basement membrane are typical of glomerulonephritis mediated by immune complexes, which are either formed locally in the glomerulus or preformed in the circulation and then deposited in the basement membranes. Such deposits occur in primary or secondary membranous nephropathy or the membranous type of glomerulonephritis of systemic lupus erythematosus. See Chapter 16.

30. **The answer is C.** *Cardiac rupture.* Cardiac rupture is a rare complication of transmural myocardial infarct found in 1% to 5% of all patients. See Chapter 11.

31. **The answer is E.** *Cirrhosis.* All the diseases listed except cirrhosis cause hyperlipidemia and predispose to or accelerate the development of atherosclerosis. See Chapter 10.

32. **The answer is E.** *Migratory thrombophlebitis.* Migratory thrombophlebitis is not a feature of cirrhosis. To the contrary, cirrhosis is associated with a bleeding tendency, because the pathologically altered liver cannot produce adequate amounts of clotting factors. See Chapter 14.

33. **The answer is B.** *Carcinoma of the rectum.* The rectum does not participate in the absorption of nutrients, and diseases of that organ do not cause malabsorption. All the other diseases cause malabsorption. See Chapter 13.

34. **The answer is E.** *Paradoxical embolism.* Except for paradoxical embolism, all the conditions listed are complications of hypertension. Paradoxical embolism refers to the passage of thromboemboli from the right heart to the left heart through an open foramen ovale or an atrial or ventricular septal defect. These venous thrombi embolize to the arterial circulation and occlude peripheral arteries in the brain, kidneys, or extremities. See Chapters 7, 10, and 12.

35. **The answer is C.** *Marked by elevated serum creatine kinase.* Myotonic dystrophy, similar to muscular dystrophies, is characterized by wasting of muscles, which is associated with an elevation of serum creatine kinase (CK), released from degenerating muscle fibers. See Chapter 27.

36. **The answer is E.** *Epithelial crescents in two-thirds of the glomeruli.* Epithelial crescents are typical of crescentic glomerulonephritis, which occurs in several forms of rapidly progressive glomerulonephritis. They are not characteristic of membranoproliferative glomerulonephritis, which is a chronic, slowly progressive disease. Membranoproliferative glomerulonephritis is characterized by proliferation of mesangial cells and reduplication of basement membranes. It is therefore known as mesan-

gioproliferative or membranoproliferative glomerulonephritis. See Chapter 16.

37. **The answer is C.** *Causes stenosis of the common bile duct.* Stenosis of the common bile duct is not a feature of primary biliary cirrhosis, which is an autoimmune disease characterized by antimitochondrial antibodies and hepatic fibrosis. It is more common in women than in men. Stenosis of the extrahepatic bile ducts occurs in some cases of primary sclerosing cholangitis, a disease that is more common in men than in women and is not associated with antimitochondrial antibodies. See Chapter 14.

38. **The answer is C.** *Eye.* Melanoma is the most common tumor of the eye in adults. See Chapter 29.

39. **The answer is B.** *Fatty change of hepatocytes.* Decreased synthesis of lipoproteins in chronic alcoholism results in fat accumulation in hepatocytes. Lipids are normally exported from the liver in the form of lipoproteins. If the apoprotein component of these molecules is not produced in adequate amounts, lipid accumulates in the liver, causing fatty liver. See Chapter 14.

40. **The answer is A.** *Ulcerative colitis.* Ulcerative colitis usually presents with rectal lesions, which spread proximally until, in late stages of the disease, the entire large intestine is finally involved. Skip lesions and involvement of the proximal colon are more typical of Crohn disease. See Chapter 13.

41. **The answer is E.** *Intraductal mucous plugs in the small pancreatic ducts.* Intraductal mucous plugs are not a feature of acute pancreatitis. Such lesions are typical of cystic fibrosis, which affects the secretion of mucus and causes obstructive lesions and chronic pancreatic insufficiency. See Chapter 15.

42. **The answer is B.** *Pancreas.* The symptoms listed reflect the secretion of vasoactive intestinal peptide by islet cell tumors (Verner-Morrison syndrome). See Chapter 15.

43. **The answer is B.** *Myocarditis.* All the other pathologic findings are common in SLE, but myocarditis is uncommon. Libman-Sacks endocarditis is the typical heart lesion of SLE. See Chapters 4 and 11.

44. **The answer is A.** *Squamous cell carcinoma of bronchus.* Squamous cell carcinoma, similar to the normal squamous epithelium of the skin, can secrete the parathyroid hormone-related peptide (PTHrP) and cause hypercalcemia. Such hypercalcemia is the most common paraneoplastic syndrome in patients with squamous cell carcinoma of the bronchus. See Chapter 12.

45. **The answer is E.** *Leydig cell tumor.* Except for Leydig cell tumors, all the other tumors contain neuroendocrine granules. Neuroendocrine granules are visible by electron microscopy in all tumors that contain polypeptide hormones, such as insulin, or biogenic amines, such as epinephrine. Leydig cell tumors secrete steroid hormones, which are not stored in the tumor cell cytoplasm or packaged into granules for secretion. See Chapters 17 and 21.

46. **The answer is C.** *Asthma.* Except for asthma, all the other lesions are possible complications of exposure to asbestos. See Chapters 8 and 12.

47. The answer is E. *Pernicious anemia.* All the conditions listed, except for pernicious anemia, predispose to or cause esophagitis. Pernicious anemia is a consequence of atrophic gastritis and is unrelated to esophagitis. See Chapter 13.

48. The answer is B. *Polycystic renal disease.* Hypertension in middle-aged people with bilaterally enlarged kidneys is usually a sign of the autosomal dominant polycystic kidney disease (ADPKD). Chronic glomerulonephritis or pyelonephritis usually causes loss of renal parenchyma, resulting in kidneys that are smaller than normal. Amyloidosis, which may cause bilateral kidney enlargement, is rare, especially in 35-year-old men. ADPKD accounts for 10% to 15% of all cases of end-stage kidney disease referred to hospitals for renal transplantation. See Chapter 16.

49. The answer is A. *Diabetes.* Nephrotic syndrome of diabetes does not have the features of membranous nephropathy, an immune-mediated glomerular disease typically found in the other conditions listed. See Chapter 16.

50. The answer is A. *Corticosteroids.* The administration of corticosteroids may cause peptic ulcers. Peptic ulcers are well-known complications of endogenous hypersecretion of corticosteroids (Cushing syndrome) or corticosteroid treatment of asthma, nephrotic syndrome, rheumatoid arthritis, and so on. See Chapters 13 and 21.

51. The answer is E. *Hyperlipidemia.* Hyperlipidemia is not a feature of acute poststreptococcal glomerulonephritis, whereas all the other findings listed are usually present. Hyperlipidemia is a feature of nephrotic syndrome, which may develop several weeks and even months after the onset of the disease. See Chapter 16.

52. The answer is A. *Granulomas.* Berylliosis is a hypersensitivity reaction to beryllium characterized by the formation of granulomas, which are indistinguishable from those of sarcoidosis. See Chapter 12.

53. The answer is D. *Circle of Willis.* Berry aneurysms of the circle of Willis are the most common aneurysms related to a congenital weakness of the vessel wall. The aneurysms occur at the base of the brain at the site at which the blood vessels originating from the carotid artery fuse with the terminal branches of the basilar artery. See Chapter 28.

54. The answer is E. *Colon cancer.* Adenocarcinoma of the colon, similar to mucinous cystadenocarcinoma of the ovary, is typically composed of mucinous cells. The other tumors listed do not produce mucin. See Chapters 13 and 18.

55. The answer is A. *Acromegaly.* Acromegaly is typically caused by a pituitary adenoma that secretes growth hormone. It grows within the sella turcica and may cause its expansion. See Chapter 21.

56. The answer is D. *Syphilis.* Gumma, a type of granuloma with central ischemic necrosis, which also contains plasma cells, is a typical feature of tertiary syphilis. It may involve any organ in the body. See Chapter 9.

57. The answer is D. *Sickle cell anemia.* Splenomegaly is found in hematopoietic malignancies and spherocytosis. In chronic sickle cell anemia, the spleen is actually very small, because sickling crises typically cause infarcts, which heal by scarring and thus destroy the spleen. The loss of splenic parenchyma is known as autosplenectomy. See Chapter 20.

58. **The answer is E.** *Initially, the shunting of blood through the defect is almost always right to left.*

59. **The answer is C.** *The peak incidence occurs between the ages of 20 and 30.* All the statements about cervical carcinoma except for C are true. The peak incidence of cervical carcinoma is in the 40- to 50-year age group. Young women rarely develop invasive cervical carcinoma, although in the age group under 30 years, cervical intraepithelial neoplasia (CIN) predominates. In untreated women, it usually takes 10 to 15 years for CIN to progress to invasive carcinoma. See Chapter 18.

60. **The answer is E.** *Trichomonas vaginalis infection.* Except for *Trichomonas vaginalis* infection, all other conditions listed may cause infertility. See Chapters 17 and 18.

61. **The answer is B.** *Endometriosis of the fallopian tube.* Endometriosis of the fallopian tubes is a lesion composed of endometrial glands and stroma, which is implanted on the serosal surface of the peritoneum covering the external surface of the tubes. Such foci enlarge upon estrogenic stimulation during the first (proliferative) half of the menstrual cycle. At the time of menstruation, foci of endometriosis undergo bleeding that is equivalent to that in the uterus. See Chapter 18.

62. **The answer is E.** *Endocarditis of the tricuspid valve.* All the conditions listed except for mitral insufficiency cause pulmonary hypertension, the cause of *cor pulmonale.* The latter term is used to describe right-sided heart failure caused by a variety of conditions that are marked by pulmonary hypertension and right ventricular hypertrophy. See Chapter 11.

63. **The answer is E.** *Hydrosalpinx.* All the other conditions listed here except for hydrosalpinx may cause vaginal bleeding. Hydrosalpinx represents the accumulation of fluid in the fallopian tube, which is atypically occluded at both ends, owing to adhesions caused by chronic inflammation and scarring. See Chapter 18.

64. **The answer is E.** *Responds favorably to hormonal therapy.* All the other statements except for E are correct. Prostatic carcinoma responds poorly to hormonal or other therapies, although the symptoms of metastases may be alleviated. See Chapter 17.

65. **The answer is C.** *Uterus.* The uterus is more often involved by primary than metastatic tumors. By contrast, metastatic tumors are more common than primary ones in the liver, lungs, adrenals, and mediastinal lymph nodes. See Chapters 12, 14, and 18.

66. **The answer is E.** *α-1-antitrypsin deficiency.* Hyperplasia of bronchial glands occurs in all the listed conditions except for α-1-antitrypsin deficiency, which is typically associated with emphysema. See Chapter 12.

67. **The answer is D.** *Liver.* Polyps occur on the skin and the luminal surface of hollow organs, but not in solid organs such as the liver. See Chapter 5.

68. **The answer is A.** *Herpesvirus.* Herpesvirus causes nuclear changes, such as eosinophilic or slightly basophilic ground-glass nuclear inclusions, Cowdry type I inclusions, or multinucleated giant cells. See Chapters 18 and 30.

69. **The answer is B.** *Silicosis.* Fibrotic nodules of silicosis contain birefringent silica crystals. These crystals are not visible by routine microscopy but can be seen under polarized light. See Chapter 12.

70. **The answer is E.** *Pernicious anemia.* All the listed conditions except for pernicious anemia are associated with an increased incidence of peptic ulcer. Pernicious anemia is a complication of atrophic gastritis, characterized by achlorhydria rather than hyperchlorhydria. The latter is a hallmark of conditions that predispose to peptic ulcer formation. See Chapter 13.

71. **The answer is A.** *Hemophilus influenzae.* Neonatal meningitis is most often caused by *Hemophilus influenzae.* See Chapter 28.

72. **The answer is C.** *Hypertension.* Hemorrhage in the internal capsule and basal ganglia of the brain is a typical complication of hypertension. See Chapter 28.

73. **The answer is E.** *Invasion of cranial bones.* All other features listed are typical of glioblastoma multiforme. These primary malignant brain tumors do not invade the cranial bones. Of all primary intracranial tumors, only meningiomas invade the cranial bones. See Chapter 28.

74. **The answer is C.** *Hyperglobulinemia.* Hyperviscosity of blood is a feature of hyperglobulinemia, as found in multiple myeloma and Waldenstrom macroglobulinemia. See Chapter 20.

75. **The answer is C.** *End-stage Paget disease of bone.* All the other conditions listed cause osteopenia (i.e., loss of bone substance). By contrast, Paget disease is characterized by osteosclerosis. In end-stage Paget disease, the sclerotic bone consists of broad osteons, separated from one another by dense bluish seams, imparting to the bone a geographic pattern. See Chapter 26.

76. **The answer is B.** *Autosomal dominant inheritance.* Huntington disease is a dementia inherited as an autosomal dominant trait. Although it is a hereditary disease, its symptoms begin in mid- to late adulthood. See Chapters 6 and 28.

77. **The answer is C.** *Caseous necrosis.* Caseous necrosis is a typical feature of granulomas caused by *M. tuberculosis.* However, caseous necrosis is not pathognomonic of tuberculosis, since it may occur in granulomas caused by many fungi such as *Cryptococcus* or *Histoplasma.* See Chapters 1, 12, and 29.

78. **The answer is D.** *Sigmoid colon.* Volvulus (i.e., twisting of an intestinal loop around itself) occurs most often in parts of the intestines that are mobile, such as the sigmoid colon or the small intestines. See Chapter 13.

79. **The answer is A.** *Increase in nasal tissue.* Hay fever is mediated by IgE, which is concentrated in the affected tissue. IgE molecules are attached to the surface of mast cells in the nasal mucosa. See Chapter 4.

80. **The answer is D.** *Goodpasture syndrome.* All the diseases listed except for Goodpasture syndrome are more common in women than in men. In Goodpasture syndrome, the male-to-female ratio is 4:1. See Chapter 16.

81. **The answer is A.** *Becker muscular dystrophy.* Becker dystrophy and Duchenne dystrophy are caused by deletions or mutations of the same gene on the X-chromosome. However, Becker dystrophy presents later in life and with milder symptoms than Duchenne dystrophy. See Chapter 27.

82. **The answer is C.** *Clostridium difficile.* Patchy necrosis of colonic mucosa covered with crusts of fibrin and cell detritus admixed to mucus are typ-

ical features of pseudomembranous colitis, which is characteristically caused by *Clostridium difficile*. See Chapter 13.

83. **The answer is C.** *Acoustic nerve.* Benign tumors in the cerebellopontine angle are most often schwannomas of the acoustic (VIII cranial) nerve. These tumors may be a feature of neurofibromatosis type II, an autosomal dominant disease. See Chapter 28.

84. **The answer is E.** *Laminar necrosis of the cerebral cortex.* All the listed lesions except for laminar necrosis are typical of multiple sclerosis. Laminar necrosis is a feature of hypotensive shock and cerebral ischemia due to hypoperfusion. See Chapter 28.

85. **The answer is B.** *Lymphocytic infiltrates in perivascular Virchow-Robin spaces.* Viral encephalitis is characterized by lymphocytic infiltrates in the perivascular Virchow-Robin spaces. See Chapter 28.

86. **The answer is D.** *Papillary necrosis of the kidney.* Papillary necrosis of the kidney is a complication of diabetes. See Chapter 16.

87. **The answer is B.** *Migratory thrombophlebitis.* All the findings listed are found in chronic myelogenous leukemia except for migratory thrombophlebitis. Leukemias are characterized by a bleeding tendency rather than thrombosis. Migratory thrombophlebitis is found in patients with carcinomas, typically carcinoma of the pancreas. See Chapter 20.

88. **The answer is E.** *Galactorrhea-amenorrhea.* Galactorrhea-amenorrhea is not a feature of fibrocystic change of the breast, whereas all other histologic findings are typical of this breast disorder. Galactorrhea-amenorrhea is a typical feature of hyperprolactinemia caused by pituitary prolactinomas. See Chapter 19.

89. **The answer is A.** *Are malignant.* Most testicular tumors are malignant. These tumors have a peak incidence in the 30- to 40-year age group. Most tumors have no hormonal activity and present as a local intrascrotal mass, rather than as distant metastases. Metastases typically occur through the lymphatics and present as lymph node enlargement in the abdomen. See Chapter 17.

90. **The answer is A.** *Hypertension.* Both Cushing syndrome and pheochromocytoma may present with hypertension. In Cushing syndrome the hypertension is caused by an excess of steroids, which cause retention of sodium and water. By contrast, pheochromocytomas secrete epinephrine, norepinephrine, or both, which cause constriction of arterioles and therefore hypertension. See Chapter 21.

91. **The answer is C.** *Metastatic carcinoma.* Primary bone tumors are rare in the elderly. Until proven otherwise, all bone tumors of the elderly should be considered metastatic. See Chapter 26.

92. **The answer is B.** *Autoimmunity.* Hyperthyroidism is most often caused by autoimmune diseases, such as Graves disease or Hashimoto disease. See Chapter 21.

93. **The answer is C.** *Pseudocyst.* A cystic cavity of the pancreas filled with turbid brownish yellow fluid is most likely a pseudocyst that has developed as a complication of acute pancreatitis. See Chapter 15.

94. **The answer is D.** *Are rich in terminal deoxynucleotidyl transferase.* All the features listed except for D are typical of Reed-Sternberg cells. Terminal

deoxynucleotidyl transferase is an enzyme typically found in immature lymphoid cells and cells of acute lymphoblastic leukemia. See Chapter 20.

95. **The answer is D.** *Raynaud disease.* All the conditions listed except for Raynaud disease increase venous pressure in the legs and predispose to the formation of varicose veins. Raynaud disease is characterized by spastic contraction of arterioles and hypoperfusion of tissues. See Chapter 10.

96. **The answer is B.** *Left ventricular hypertrophy.* All the changes listed, except for left ventricular hypertrophy, are typical features of mitral stenosis. The left ventricle receives less blood than normal; thus there is no left ventricular hypertrophy. See Chapter 11.

97. **The answer is D.** *Ankylosing spondylitis.* All the features listed except for ankylosing spondylitis are typical of rheumatic fever. Ankylosing spondylitis is a disease of unknown etiology and is not related to rheumatic fever. See Chapter 26.

98. **The answer is A.** *Hypertension.* Stenosis of a renal artery causes renal ischemia and stimulates secretion of renin, which acts on angiotensinogen and causes hypertension. See Chapter 16.

99. **The answer is B.** *Nephrosclerosis due to artherosclerosis.* Loss of renal parenchyma in the elderly is most often related to ischemia caused by atherosclerosis. The term *nephrosclerosis* describes the small fibrotic kidney that has undergone scarring due to ischemia. See Chapter 16.

100. **The answer is C.** *Craniopharyngioma.* Craniopharyngiomas are tumors of the sellar region and are typically located above the tentorium, which is interposed between the cerebrum and the cerebellum. Medulloblastoma and cerebellar astrocytomas are by definition subtentorial tumors, because they originate in the cerebellum. Schwannomas occur in the cerebellopontine angle, which is also subtentorial. Meningiomas may occur in both subtentorial and supratentorial compartments of the cranium. See Chapter 38.

101. **The answer is C.** *Medulloblastoma.* All the tumors listed except for medulloblastoma can occur in the cerebrum or the spinal cord. Medulloblastomas arise only in the cerebellum. See Chapter 28.

Final Practical Photographic Examination

Questions

DIRECTIONS: The questions in this examination relate to the color photographs beginning on page 243. Study each photograph and answer the corresponding question by choosing the single best answer.

_____ 1. This tumor is a
A. chondrosarcoma.
B. rhabdomyosarcoma.
C. squamous cell carcinoma.
D. transitional cell carcinoma.
E. teratoma.

_____ 2. This duodenal lesion is typically associated with
A. achlorhydria.
B. pernicious anemia.
C. melena.
D. insulinoma.
E. jaundice.

_____ 3. What is the most likely diagnosis for this intestinal lesion?
A. Tubular adenoma
B. Villous adenoma
C. Hyperplastic polyp
D. Inflammatory polyp
E. Sarcoma

_____ 4. This salivary gland lesion causes
A. keratomalacia.
B. seborrheic keratosis.
C. xerostomia.
D. suppurative staladenitis.
E. oral leukoplakia.

_____ 5. What is the most likely diagnosis for this nasal lesion?
A. Olfactory neuroblastoma
B. Inverted papilloma
C. Squamous papilloma
D. Lethal midline granuloma
E. Juvenile angiofibroma

_____ **6.** The enzyme histochemical reaction for demonstrating ATPase was applied to this muscle biopsy. These findings are most consistent with the diagnosis of
   A. polymyositis.
   B. Duchenne muscular dystrophy.
   C. neurologic atrophy with reinervation.
   D. myasthenia gravis.
   E. myositis ossificans.

_____ **7.** The muscle disease illustrated in this photograph is best classified as
   A. metabolic.
   B. congenital.
   C. genetic.
   D. autoimmune.
   E. neurogenic.

_____ **8.** This cervical "pap" smear shows changes indicative of
   A. carcinoma in situ.
   B. invasive carcinoma.
   C. herpesvirus infection.
   D. papillomavirus infection.
   E. *Trichomonas vaginalis* infection.

_____ **9.** The ovarian tumor originated from
   A. germinal epithelium.
   B. germ cells.
   C. sex cord cells.
   D. nonspecific ovarian stroma.
   E. ovarian hilar cells.

_____ **10.** This intrathoracic tumor is a
   A. lobular carcinoma.
   B. mucinous (gelatinous) adenocarcinoma.
   C. tubular carcinoma.
   D. mesothelioma.
   E. Paget disease.

_____ **11.** This photograph of a glomerulus is most consistent with the diagnosis of
   A. proliferative glomerulonephritis.
   B. crescentic glomerulonephritis.
   C. focal and segmental sclerosis with hyalinosis.
   D. lipoid nephrosis.
   E. Kimmelstiel-Wilson disease.

_____ **12.** This patient was a 30-year-old, tall man, with subluxation of the lens who died within minutes of developing excruciating chest pain. The most likely cause of death was
   A. ruptured left ventricular aneurysm.
   B. dissecting aneurysm of the aorta.
   C. myocardial infarct.
   D. coronary embolism.
   E. mitral stenosis.

_____ **13.** This disease is inherited as a(n)
  A. polygenic trait.
  B. autosomal dominant trait.
  C. autosomal recessive trait.
  D. sex-linked dominant trait.
  E. sex-linked recessive trait.

_____ **14.** This brain lesion is in most instances a complication of
  A. congenital cerebral malformation.
  B. inborn error of metabolism.
  C. circulatory disturbance.
  D. malignancy.
  E. multiple sclerosis.

_____ **15.** The lesion illustrated in this immunofluorescence photomicrograph of a glomerulus is typically associated with
  A. gross hematuria.
  B. microscopic hematuria.
  C. proteinuria.
  D. glycosuria.
  E. papillary necrosis.

_____ **16.** This testicular tumor is typically
  A. radiosensitive.
  B. bilateral.
  C. a tumor of old age.
  D. hormonally active.
  E. common before puberty.

_____ **17.** This malignant lung tumor is
  A. derived from type I pneumocytes.
  B. hormonally active.
  C. an adenocarcinoma.
  D. inoperable.
  E. more common in men than in women.

_____ **18.** Which of the following is an important complication of this cardiac lesion?
  A. Cerebral abscess
  B. Tubulointerstitial nephritis
  C. Hydronephrosis
  D. Hepatitis
  E. Cirrhosis

_____ **19.** This pulmonary lesion is caused by
  A. viruses.
  B. bacteria.
  C. toxic fumes.
  D. oxygen toxicity.
  E. asbestos.

_____ **20.** Tumors of the same histologic type as this skin tumor may also originate in the
A. brain.
B. bronchi.
C. liver.
D. muscle.
E. eye.

_____ **21.** This finding is diagnostic of
A. Burkitt lymphoma.
B. Sezary syndrome.
C. Hodgkin's disease.
D. chronic myelogenous leukemia.
E. agranulocytosis.

_____ **22.** This type of malignancy occurs most often in the
A. long bones of young people of either sex.
B. long bones of elderly men.
C. short hand bones of children.
D. short bones of extremities of elderly women.
E. skull bones.

_____ **23.** The best serum marker for this liver tumor is
A. alkaline phosphatase.
B. acid phosphatase.
C. alanine aminotransferase.
D. creatine kinase.
E. a-fetoprotein.

_____ **24.** This liver lesion represents
A. hepatocellular carcinoma.
B. cholangiocellular carcinoma.
C. bile duct hamartoma.
D. metastatic carcinoma.
E. cirrhosis with a malignant tumor that could be either primary or metastatic.

A n s w e r s

1. **The answer is B.** This photograph illustrates a rhabdomyosarcoma. Note the striation of malignant rhabdomyoblasts.

2. **The answer is C.** This photograph illustrates a duodenal peptic ulcer. Melena is a common finding in patients with bleeding peptic ulcer.

3. **The answer is A.** This is a pedunculated tumor of the colon. Most of these tumors are tubular adenomas.

4. **The answer is C.** This photograph shows a massive lymphoid infiltrate and epimyoepithelial islands in a salivary gland (arrows), typical of Sjögren syndrome. Xerostomia (dry mouth) is a typical symptom that develops because of destruction of salivary gland tissue.

5. **The answer is E.** This tumor is a juvenile angiofibroma composed of cellular fibrous tissue and prominent blood vessels.

6. **The answer is D.** This photograph shows pale type I fibers and dark type II fibers intermixed in a normal checkerboard pattern. These findings are most consistent with myasthenia gravis, a disease in which the normal muscle morphology is preserved. All other diseases listed are associated with typical histopathologic changes.

7. **The answer is D.** This photograph shows skeletal muscle infiltrated by mononuclear inflammatory cells, typical of polymyositis. Polymositis responds well to corticosteroid therapy and is considered an autoimmune disease.

8. **The answer is C.** This cervical smear shows features typical of herpesvirus infection, including multinucleated cells, and nuclei that have a "ground-glass" appearance.

9. **The answer is C.** This photograph shows an ovarian granuloma tumor, which originates from sex cord cells. The cells are arranged in a follicular pattern, forming so-called Call-Exner bodies.

10. **The answer is D.** This photograph shows a tumor composed of epithelial cells lining tissue clefts and spindle cells forming bundles. This biphasic composition is typical of mesothelioma.

11. **The answer is A.** This photograph illustrates the changes typical of diffuse proliferative glomerulonephritis. An increased number of cells can be seen in all mesangial areas and capillary loops; thus the lesion is diffuse rather than segmental. There are no signs of sclerosis, necrosis, or crescent formation.

12. **The answer is B.** This photograph shows arachnodactyly. In combination with subluxation of the lens, this finding is highly suggestive of Marfan syndrome. Dissecting aneurysm is a common cause of sudden death in these patients.

13. **The answer is B.** This photograph shows multiple skin neurofibromas typical of neurofibromatosis type 1, which is an autosomal dominant disease.

14. **The answer is C.** This photograph shows a cystic infarct of the brain, which is in most cases a complication of atherosclerosis and other circulatory disturbances that cause cerebral ischemia.

15. **The answer is C.** The "lumpy-bumpy" granular pattern of immunofluorescence of glomerular basement membranes is typical of membranous nephropathy, which presents with proteinuria and nephrotic syndrome.

16. **The answer is A.** This photograph shows a seminoma, which is a radiosensitive testicular tumor usually curable by surgery combined with radiotherapy. The peak incidence of seminoma occurs at 40 years of age. This tumor does not occur before puberty and is rarely bilateral.

17. **The answer is C.** This microphotograph shows an adenocarcinoma. Note the irregular glandlike structures typical of this malignancy. These tumors originate from bronchial cells and are not hormonally active. They may be operable if diagnosed early and are less common in men.

18. **The answer is A.** This photograph shows infectious endocarditis. Emboli of infected material from the cardiac valves may cause cerebral abscesses.

19. **The answer is B.** This photograph shows polymorphonuclear leukocytes in the alveoli and bronchi, a typical feature of bacterial pneumonia.

20. **The answer is B.** This photograph shows a squamous cell carcinoma, the most common histologic type of bronchogenic carcinoma.

21. **The answer is C.** This photograph shows a Reed-Sternberg cell, which is a diagnostic hallmark of Hodgkin's disease.

22. **The answer is A.** This photograph illustrates the histologic features of osteosarcoma. Between malignant cells (osteoblasts) are lamellae of osteoid and partially calcified and newly formed bony trabeculae. This tumor occurs most often in long bones of young persons and does not show any sex predilection.

23. **The answer is E.** These photographs show a hepatocellular carcinoma. Alpha-fetoprotein (AFP) is the best serum marker for primary liver cancer.

24. **The answer is E.** This slide shows a liver studded with numerous nodules typical of metastatic carcinoma. There is no evidence of cirrhosis.

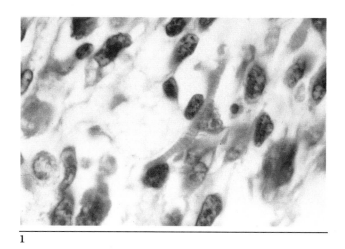

1

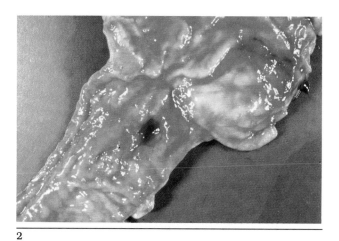

2

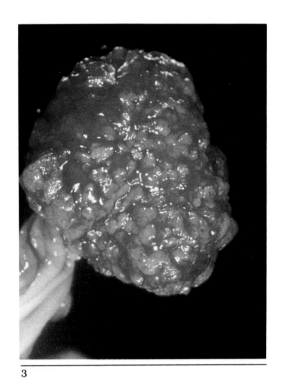

3

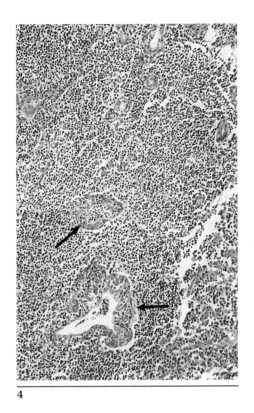

4

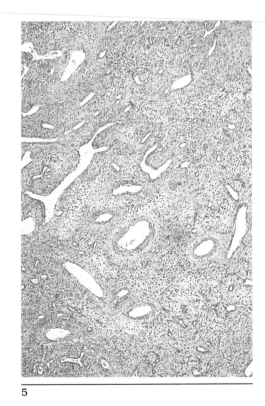

5

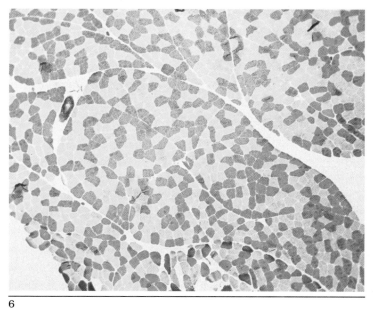

6

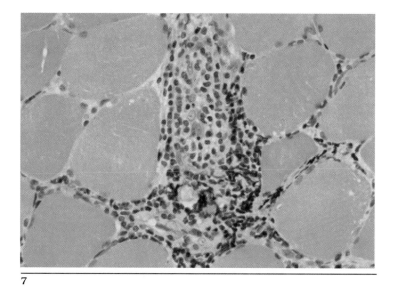

7

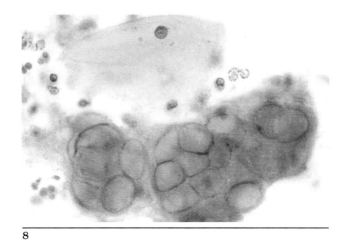

8

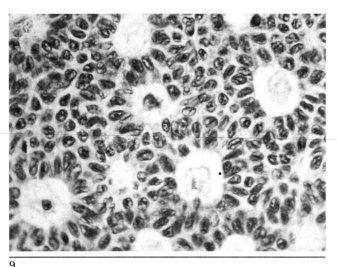

9

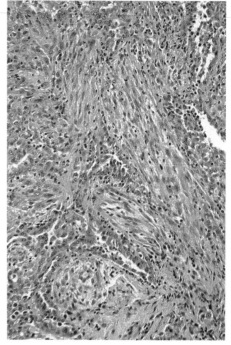

10

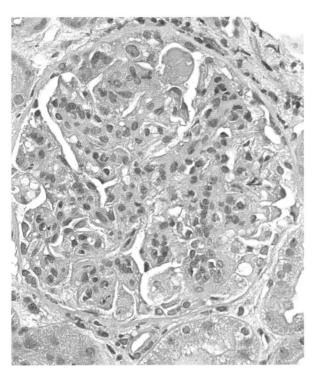

11

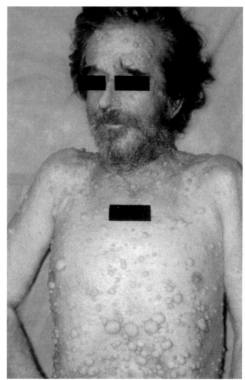

13

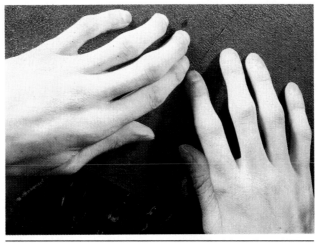

12

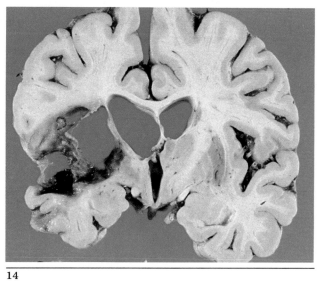

14

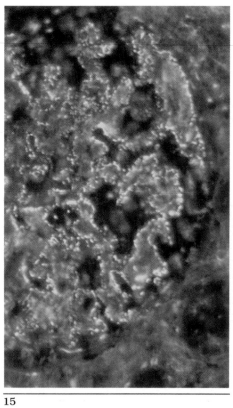

15

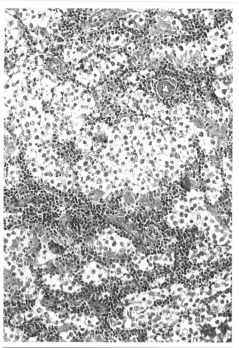

16

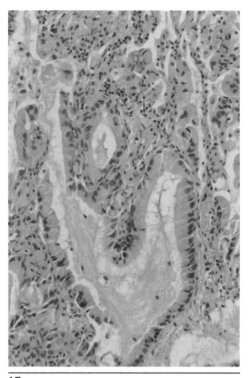

17

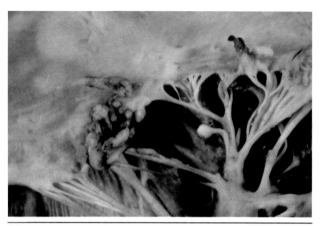

18

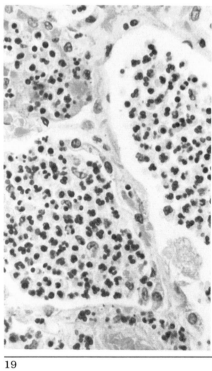

19

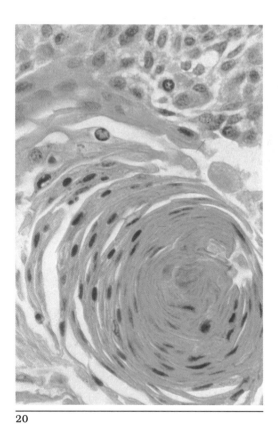

20

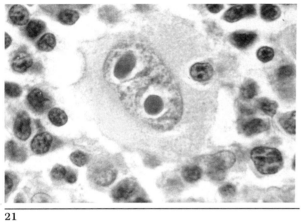

21

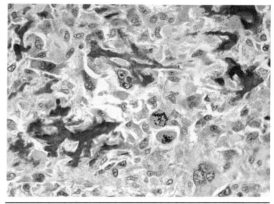

22

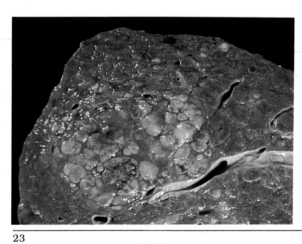

23

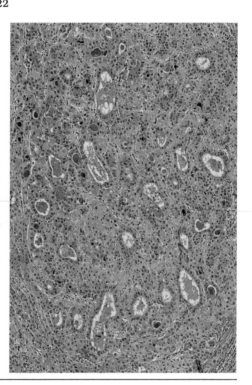

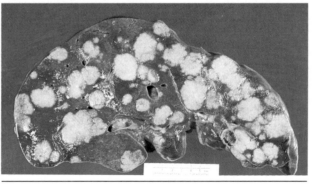

24